A QUIET ROAR

Caitlin Press Inc.
8100 Alderwood Road, Halfmoon Bay, BC V0N 1Y1
www.caitlin-press.com
Text and cover design by Vici Johnstone
Printed in Canada

Caitlin Press Inc. acknowledges financial support from the Government of Canada and the Canada Council for the Arts, and the Province of British Columbia through the British Columbia Arts Council and the Book Publisher's Tax Credit.

| Canada Council for the Arts Conseil des Arts du Canada | BRITISH COLUMBIA ARTS COUNCIL | Funded by the Government of Canada | Canada |

Library and Archives Canada Cataloguing in Publication
Redl, Heidi, 1962-, author
    A quiet roar : living with multiple sclerosis / Heidi Redl.
ISBN 978-1-987915-37-2 (softcover)
        1. Redl, Heidi, 1962-. 2. Multiple sclerosis—Patients—Canada—
Biography. I. Title.
RC377.R43 2017   362.196'8340092   C2016-907719-5

A Quiet Roar

Living with Multiple Sclerosis

Heidi Redl

CAITLIN PRESS

This book is dedicated to my children: Ben, Sam and Lexie.
It is also dedicated to all the people who are fighting MS
right along with me.

CONTENTS

My Peculiar Path

When you come to a fork in the road, take it.
—Yogi Berra

The highway sloped down and curved gently to the right when I heard myself break the silence in the car. "If it's a brain tumour and its removal would mean I become a vegetable, I don't want it removed. I'd rather die than be a vegetable."

"Let's just take it one step at a time and see what the doc says," Tom answered calmly. Then he added, "I get where you're coming from, though."

It was 2004. My husband Tom and I were driving down to Kamloops from our ranch home in Miocene for an appointment with a neurologist. It was a beautiful May day and through the car windows I could see thickly treed hills with patches of rolling grassland on their sides and in meadows at their feet, the same grassland patches I used to ride my horse Lucky over. I hadn't been riding for more than a year but I still dreamt and even daydreamt about riding, and today an imaginary black horse galloped along beside our car, racing over the hills and fields in the sunshine with me clinging tightly to its back. My daydream world was quite different from my reality. The past year had actually been spent searching for answers to the question of why I suddenly couldn't walk with a normal gait.

My left leg dragged and my left foot dropped, until I would trip over my own toes. Added to that, I was always exhausted.

"It will be better to know what the problem is," I said, but I didn't know if I really believed that.

Tom nodded in agreement. "It will be good to know what we're dealing with."

Mile after mile flowed by. On both sides of the car, summer was slowly coming to the Cariboo, our area of BC. While Tom eyed up the hayfields and wondered aloud when the "first cut" would happen, I looked at the same hayfields with a rather more jaundiced eye and wondered quietly if I would be alive to see another harvest.

We arrived in Kamloops and went together to a floor in the hospital where I would undergo preliminary tests before my appointment with the neurologist. The tests were unpleasant. A nurse attached electrodes to my feet. The sharp stings when they fired were not nearly as hard to stand as the nurse herself, who was obnoxiously cheerful.

She insisted on telling us about her horses and her love-ly horseback rides. It was as if she was rubbing salt in a wound. Riding horses had been impossible to do for the last year. Maybe now it was no longer possible, forever.

"Everything is normal here," the nurse chirped with a smile, tugging off the electrodes. I sensed right away that this was not good news. If my nerves in my legs are nor-mal, I knew, that meant the problem *was* in my brain.

When the nurse finally left, Tom and I waited in the examining room for the neurologist to come. I still sat on the examining table in the green hospital gown and Tom moved to stand beside me. I think he put his hand on my shoulder but I was too nervous to respond. The room smelled of disinfectant, sharp and noxious. The smell added to the ill feeling swirling through my gut and my head. When he came in, the serious-faced neurologist ran through some more tests with me: touching my finger to my nose, repeatedly, flexing each finger, and so on, ad nauseum. With each test, I could see the evidence of some sort of brain injury mounting. My left hand didn't move as quickly and surely as my right hand, I stumbled when I walked to the door across the room, and my eyes moved like windshield wipers as they followed Dr. Mosewich's pen across my field of vision, one lagging behind the other as they no longer moved smoothly together.

Finally, when I could not physically do another test without vomiting from fear, Dr. Mosewich sat down on a stool and faced me where I was perched on the edge of the examining table.

"What do you think it is?" he asked me gently.

"I think it's multiple sclerosis."

He raised his hands, palms upward, let them drop back in his lap and with a rueful smile said, "I don't like to drop bombs on people. I think you're right though. How did you know?"

I thought about it. I had actually known for a while. True, I hadn't known the specific name of the disease on my own, but I knew it was something serious that was wrong with me. Since that day, I've learned that people with multiple sclerosis often know that something is wrong in their bodies for years before the first symptoms show up and usually by the time we get to a neurologist, the diagnosis only confirms what we already knew.

In my case, I had "known" since the night I dreamt of the airplane crash, more than ten years before. In my dream I was standing on the road by Rose Lake on a brilliantly sunny day, looking up the hill when a large white airplane emblazoned with red letters spelling "I AM" roared through the blue, blue sky over the treetops and then crashed into the crest of the hill. I turned to the dark green house behind me and saw a fat, old, grey-haired woman sitting in the basement eating cherry pastries. Later, still disturbed by the vividness of the dream and doing some psychological reading and research, I learned that the basement of a house signifies subconsciousness and all people you meet in your dreams are parts of your own personality. The fat, old woman sitting in the basement was me, stuffing myself with the sweets I love in defiance of the disaster unfolding in front of me. I AM signified my ego, and my ego, my sense of myself, was crashing with the advent of holes, or scleroses, appearing at random in my brain.

I had gotten the actual name "multiple sclerosis" from a physiotherapist who watched me closely while I walked down her hallway on one of my desperate searches for help back in Williams Lake.

"That's MS," she'd said. "My sister has it and she walks like you do, dragging the left leg." I know you're not supposed to shoot the messenger but nevertheless, I haven't been back to her practice since then. I haven't been able to forgive her for telling me I have MS.

It was a different matter hearing it confirmed by Dr. Mosewich when I was sitting in his office. I got to be the one to label it first. Maybe that gave me a feeling of control over the situation, even if I knew I was losing control of my body.

Multiple sclerosis. A label. I understood what it meant: my central nervous system, which runs through my spinal cord and terminates in my brain, was afflicted by an autoimmune disease. Somehow, I had drawn the genetic short straw when I was conceived. Multiple sclerosis is a disease that attacks myelin, which is the protective "fatty sheath" that covers everyone's nerves. When the myelin is attacked it becomes damaged and inflamed and because it's necessary for nerve impulses to travel along the nerve pathways in our nervous systems, even minor interruptions caused by inflammation and myelin damage will cause those impulses to fail to reach their destinations unimpeded. In the early stages of multiple sclerosis, the damage and its symptoms are slight: gait impairment (foot drop, limping) and fatigue. Later on in the disease the damage becomes more substantial and scar tissue, or scleroses, replaces the myelin. Then the nerve impulses are completely disrupted and the nerves themselves are damaged. Later symptoms include loss of walking ability entirely, difficulty swallowing, cognitive impairment and, in the worst cases, death. I had indeed drawn the genetic short straw. The symptoms I displayed in Dr. Mosewich's office already included lack of coordination, vision problems, generalized weakness, impaired sensation and I readily admitted to extreme fatigue. I had to: I was constantly yawning, even there in that doctor's office.

"Go home and forget you have it," Dr. Mosewich advised me. There is no cure, he further told me, and MS affects different people in different ways. The course the disease would take with me could be quite different than the way it affects others.

There was no way of knowing what to expect.

"I don't want you to be scared," Tom said as we left

the neurologist's office. We drove over the bridge at Savona and the bright sunlight of that beautiful day was sparkling off the deep blue water of Kamloops Lake. On such a lovely day, it was surreal and strange to contemplate the fact that I have a serious, debilitating disease.

"MS. That's hard to believe."

"I always thought you would end up looking after me as we get older. Now, it looks like I'll be looking after you." Tom was still calm, a lot calmer than I was, I think.

The car hummed along, swallowing the miles until we finally drove into Miocene and the ranch that had been our home for over fifteen years. I stared at the ranch fields, the cows, and the horses, and I wondered if I would still be able to help my husband on the ranch. Would I be able to hay in the summer and ride behind the cows as they were pushed out to range?

Now it's 2017. Since that diagnosis my primary goal for my life's journey has changed many times. In fact, I'm not sure it's nailed down yet, but I know I want to reach a place of happiness and contentment in my life. I've learned that having multiple sclerosis is primarily a mental game. I try to stay strong, try to minimize my physical losses, to be bright and upbeat while watching and sensing my strength and abilities slip away day by day like sand through my fingers. I have tried just about everything to reverse this disease and not to give up the fight. According to a timeline I've seen for people with progressive MS, nine years is the average length of time it takes for people to go from diagnosis through cane to wheelchair.

I have never been OK with being average.

CHILDHOOD AND YOUTH

One of the luckiest things that can happen to you in life is, I think, a happy childhood.
—Agatha Christie

A tall white horse features largely in my first real memory of childhood. When I was barely three years old, before my family had moved from Germany, we visited the ranch in Miocene where my father had grown up. I blame my grandfather for my lifelong addiction to horses because it was during that trip that Grampa took me for a ride on Blanco.

Blanco was a wise old horse, but he was also "barn sour," which means he would start to run towards the barn whenever he was turned around for home. That day, with the hard earth and the green summer grass flowing by under Blanco's hooves, was magical to me. It was my first ride on a horse and I was both scared at the new sensations and unbelievably excited as I sat deep in the worn leather saddle in front of Grampa. My short legs couldn't reach down to the stirrups so I had a death grip on the saddle horn with my little fingers. When Grampa turned Blanco towards the barn, he took off. Clinging to the saddle horn and then feeling my grampa's hands holding me tight in front of him, I felt safe. I wanted Blanco to go faster and faster. This was fun! It was the start of a lifelong love affair with horses. I didn't know it then but my most treasured memories of childhood and youth would all involve horses.

As for Blanco specifically, I remember him as one of those horses that "thinks." He had a few tricks to get rid of riders when he didn't want to be packing them around. His favourite trick was to walk so close to a large tree that he could "rub" the rider right out of the saddle on his back. Like me, Blanco liked to be in control. He had his own ideas of how life should be.

I have spent most of my life in the country where I first rode Blanco and then a succession of other horses, but I was born in 1962 on December 11 shortly after 8:00 am in the renowned spa city of Baden-Baden, Germany. In the neighbouring quiet, small city of Rastatt, close to the Canadian air force base where my father worked, I went to the kindergarten across the street from our apartment building starting at the age of three. That was following German traditions, where children go to kindergarten from ages three to five. It was not a good start for my education. I have hazy memories of being sent home on my first day for being bad. I threw a toy train across the room in a fit of temper. I think I must have been born with a rebel streak. The toy train incident was just one of many in those early years. I was a headstrong child, healthy and energetic, showing no sign of the devastating immune disease with which I was born.

My sister Barb was born in 1966, and the next year my father was transferred to Cold Lake, Alberta and we all moved back to Canada. I was old enough by then to know what was happening and to understand why my grandmother, Omi, was crying when we left Germany. She gave me a little cardboard pink suitcase that I treasured for years. A couple of years ago I gave it to my young niece Erin, who in many ways reminds me of myself at that age: independent and quietly headstrong. OK, stubborn as heck.

I started real school at age five in Cold Lake. I continued to challenge my parents with my independent spirit. I walked home from school by myself that winter, bundled head-to-foot in winter clothes and with my dad's thick, black, woollen scarf around my face. I remember one afternoon especially well: after a heavy snowstorm, the subdivision driveways had all been ploughed out and I gave in to the urge to climb up every single, steep pile of driveway snow and slide down the other side on my little bottom. It was pitch black and bitterly cold by the time I got home to my frantic mother.

In 1969, when I was in grade 2, Grampa died. Granny was dying of cancer and needed help so my dad quit the air force and we moved to his parents' ranch, the one he'd grown up on, in Miocene, BC. That is how I eventually grew up on a cattle ranch and why, as a young girl, I identified very much with being Canadian. My German mother firmly pushed the "German is better" point of view on everything but I was a rebellious child. Not only was I strong-willed and rebellious, I was also as Canadian as I could be. I went on youth exchanges to other parts of Canada, like PEI and Alberta, on trips promoted by our then government of Pierre Elliot Trudeau. I was active in the 4-H program, raising steer calves every year. And, of course, I rode. I was always riding horses over our ranch deep in the interior of BC.

Miocene was a small, rural, old-fashioned ranching community scattered over the heavily treed hills fifty kilometres east of Williams Lake, in the Cariboo region of central BC. When we moved there, I immediately started riding one of the big, rough, ranch geldings. Rebel was huge, probably part draft horse, and very gentle. He was bigger and faster than old Blanco, who was "semi-retired" in the pastures around the house. Since I was a big girl now, being all of seven years old, I could handle a faster horse. I rode around the ranch home pastures and in the hayfields, over the yellowed stalks when the hay was harvested or over the new, fresh green grass in the spring. My time with Rebel, combined with the smell and feel of the worn, smooth leather reins and deep, old cowboy saddle, cemented a lifelong love of the ranching lifestyle.

Of course, there were things that made ranch life difficult for our family and things that were far beyond my young understanding. Grampa was gone and we lived in the house he had lived in with Granny, who was already ill when we came. My memories of the house on the ranch are primarily of the kitchen and are of heavy, white cupboards and counters and daffodil-yellow drawers and cupboard doors. I loved that white-and-yellow combination. It was so cheerful. I would come downstairs when Granny was still alive and she would be standing at the woodstove with a red ribbon tied up in her white hair, making pancakes. She made us snowman-shaped pancakes and I thought she was absolutely clever. I didn't get to know Granny well but I do remember, with some shame, being bored out of my little mind and wanting to escape when she called me into her sickroom to visit. I had no interest in a dying old lady. Her grotesquely swollen left arm fascinated me though. It was many years before I knew Granny had died of breast cancer and was just in her fifties when she passed away. Granny died a mere thirty days after Grampa suffered a fatal heart attack and they are buried beside each other in the cemetery on the ranch.

The family house on the ranch was a true pioneer ranch home, with none of the modern fixings that rural communities have now, especially at first when money was tight as Dad tried to ranch and hold things together in the aftermath of his parents' deaths. For a short time he and his siblings flirted with the idea of ranching together but then they finally gave up and split up the ranch into individual homesteads. We kept the house, the hill behind it, and the hayfield below. Life there was a pretty rustic existence. It was a long time before we got hot running water or even an indoor toilet. The house itself was a simple square building with two stories and white board siding (which I remember repainting when I was about fifteen), and small, single-paned windows. I remember washing those windows every spring, including sitting on the porch roof to wash the upstairs bedroom windows. I also remember I sometimes crawled through my upstairs bedroom window to escape the house at night. I found lots of opportunities to exert my independence on the ranch.

The outside house walls were lined with sawdust insulation. The house was cold even during the heat of the summer but it was extremely cold from October to June. As the sawdust settled over the years, it left empty gaps in those walls where there was no insulation at all. The house did have two chimneys and two wood-burning stoves, but at minus 40 degree temperatures in December the stoves' heat made barely a dent in the bone-crushing cold. The old

McClary cookstove in the kitchen stayed there for many years after we moved in, but it wasn't too long before Mom and Dad replaced the little pot-bellied wood-burning stove in the living room with a larger wood-burning stove. Whenever I came in from playing outside in the winter, I would peel off my stiff boots and lie on the floor in front of the wood stove with my frozen feet propped up on it. When I felt little rivers of ice run up my legs towards my belly I knew the cold blood from my feet could now circulate through my body and slowly warm up and I could use my thawed-out feet again. I had usually been out tobogganing and would come in late, waiting for the sky to start darkening to deep purple and the house lights to shine warm yellow before I would leave my toboggan runs on the hill beside the house. I can remember these things clearly and I'm so glad I lived those experiences, especially now in hindsight when I can no longer climb up a hillside in the snow. Frozen feet didn't matter when I could go rushing headlong down a hill on a toboggan in the dark. That was magical and I was happy because the safe house with the warm, yellow lights was always there.

During those winters I used to stay in bed and get dressed under the covers, because it was too cold to get out of bed to put my clothes on. Every morning I would take some time to admire the glittering white patterns the frost would paint on the inside of my bedroom window. Thick frost ferns and sparkling frost leaves seemed to invite me to go outside into a magic forest world. My pragmatic side noted the ferns and forest of ice were layered on the *inside* of my window pane and that dressed as I was, with my feet protected only by socks and slippers, was no way for my body to go exploring outside. My imagination, however, tromped through those icy fern gullies and found wonderful crystal caves and palaces. I was born with a strong imagination and an artist's eye for colour and patterns. I didn't appreciate it much when I was younger, although I enjoyed using these abilities in daydreams, to make life more exciting and wonderful than it otherwise was. Now though, I am forever grateful for my imagination and artist's eye. No matter what scene I look at, I can travel through it and beyond it and my wheelchair never accompanies me on my mind's travels.

We finally got hot running water in the house when I was about nine and Barb was six. By then, Mom and Dad could afford an electric water heater in the bathroom. Hot water in the house, however, was still a luxury. The ranch well that supplied our house water was poor and so we never had enough water for each of us to have our own bath. We learned early on to save water and to be thrifty with it, as thrifty as we were with everything else. Barb and I had to share baths. First one would get to play in the bathtub, then the other. I only remember soap bubbles and warm water once. The rest of the time I remember tepid water and washing my hair under the bathtub tap. Then yanking the comb through it. We didn't know about conditioner. Maybe it wasn't even available back then.

Bath time wasn't the only time that Barb and I shared. Barb and I spent a lot of time together when we were growing up. Neighbours lived far away from us and there were very few that were our age. We were each other's only playmates and the great outdoors was our only playground. Each fall Barb and I would go outside with buckets and we would run under the trees by the garden, trying to catch the leaves as they fell. Because they were gold in colour, each leaf represented money. Each of us had a "Trading Post" by the woodpile behind the chicken house and we would spend our gold there on grass seeds and brightly coloured rocks we had collected beforehand.

I was the older sister and therefore I bossed Barb around unmercifully. She, though, was strong and stockier in build than I was and she didn't take my bossing kindly. It wasn't too many years before she could beat me at things like wrestling and I had to rely on my speed to outrun her when she was mad. Barb was born with bright red hair and a temper to match it. Board games on our living room floor were always tense as both of us wanted to win, badly, and the game would invariably end in a fight. I was careful to keep the fights in the verbal arena because I couldn't beat my little sister physically. She was too strong.

Although Barb and I had the usual sibling arguments we also shared a lot of laughter. One time I remember in particular is a night we lost power. Nothing unusual in that—we often lost power along our rural road—but this was a specific night when I was about ten and Barb was seven. Dad had a kerosene lamp that he could light and we ate a dinner that was cooked on the wood stove while Barb's copper-coloured hair shone in the glow of the kerosene lamp that sat in the middle of our supper table. Dad had a small battery-operated radio where we could listen to other people call BC Hydro and check on the progress of the outage. On that night, with the painted black Scottie dogs romping around the base of Granny's old kerosene lamp, we overheard our neighbour call BC Hydro to complain: "it's black as Toby's ass out here, except for the light of the moon."

Barb and I laughed about that, harder even when we saw that Dad was laughing too. We really had no idea what "Toby's ass" referred to; we just didn't hear swear words as kids, not even from the other kids on the school bus. Dad would come close, but stayed with "sap" or "north end of a horse going south" and the occasional "jackass." Dad probably did swear one summer day when I was eleven or so, although I forget what he called me. He must have been sick with worry. I had just confessed to drinking diesel mixture out of the old milk jug that was sitting by the hay elevator in the hayfield. I had confused the purple diesel mixture with the purple Kool-Aid drink we kept in just such a container for ourselves in the hot weather. Another neighbour advocated some obnoxious cure that would make me throw up, but Mom and Dad decided to wait it out and see what happened. I doubt I drank more than the first swallow, due to the taste of gas, but I can't, now, claim to have suffered no lasting effects. Who knows? Maybe that incident was just one more straw to push this body over the edge.

My usual childhood diet, of course, did not include diesel. We may not have had a lot of luxuries, but we were never short on food. Fresh vegetables were plentiful when I was growing up, thanks to our garden and Mom's persistent efforts to provide healthy food for us. I'm the first to admit it was often delicious too, as in the case of tomato cake. Tomato cake is what we here in Canada would call a flan, but the base is a deep, savoury, flaky pie crust. Ripe, red tomato slices are baked on top of the crust in a layer of concentric, overlapping circles on a bed of eggs and cream. In fact, the only reason I try to grow tomatoes now is in the often-vain hope I'll have enough ripe, red ones to make a tomato cake, like the one my grandmother, and then mother, used to make when I was a child. Anything I know about gardening I learned from Mom. She learned about gardening in the Cariboo from Dad's Aunt Olive and other people who had experience coaxing vegetables and flowers to grow in the tough, cold climate.

The older pioneers in the small community, most of whom were related to us, taught us a lot about living there and, by default, a lot about healthy eating. I know now that diet plays a huge role in regulating emotions and that there is a proven link between our guts and our minds or emotions. I was a healthy child and while growing up the only fruit, and ergo sugar, we got readily was from local berries. My favourite source of sugar was definitely saskatoon berries. As children, we used to go up on Rose Hill and pick saskatoons every August. There was one giant saskatoon bush, or tree, in the middle of the hill and, if we got there before the birds did, we could fill our pails easily. The saskatoons were small, almost dry, and very, very sweet.

Aunt Olive was one of the people who taught Mom, and therefore us, a lot about local foods. Thanks to her we would get dressed up in long-sleeved shirts buttoned up at the wrists, long pants over black, rubber boots with elastics cinching the pants in at the ankle, and we would carry bleach cans carved out into containers hanging from belts at our waists. The final touches were thick, woollen scarves wrapped around our heads to protect us from the mosquitoes. All of this so we could go out to Quesnel Lake and pick berries with Aunt Olive in the logging clear-cuts above the lake. Miserable in the heat of those sweltering hillsides, I had no choice but to listen as Aunt Olive would harangue me with stories about how fast she could pick at my age and how she and her mother would race each other to pick the most berries. She would tut-tut at how few blueberries or huckleberries were rolling around in the bottom of my bleach can. I would swat at the devil's club thorns, shinny over fallen cedar logs on the forest floor, watch for black bears and generally avoid Aunt Olive and the mosquitoes as much as possible. I hated berry-picking. Although blueberries and huckleberries were delicious, the effort to collect them didn't seem quite worth it when I was young.

Olive's husband Uncle Bill came out with us once or twice and he was fun. He would tell stories about the time he was picking on one side of a huge blueberry bush and when he got it done and went around to the other side he found a black bear picking those same berries. He claimed he and the bear each went up a different tree then and just waited each other out. Besides Uncle Bill, a pleasant find in the thick woods and head-high devil's club would be the odd twenty-one-metre fallen cedar tree. I would hoist myself up on one end and, balancing easily, would glory in being able to walk its length free from the underbrush that tore at my clothes and skin down below on the forest floor. My strong, young body provided me with many hours of thoughtless pleasure but none more so than when I was climbing something. I loved to climb and turned many a fallen log or pile of rocks into a mountaineering adventure, thanks to my imagination and a great sense of balance. To this day, I cannot drive past a mountain without experiencing the urge to climb it. I think that comes from growing up in the Cariboo, in sight of the mountains.

The outside world hardly reached us in Miocene, and still barely penetrates the mountains today. When I was a kid, global communication was near-impossible and local communication was not a whole lot easier. We started out on a party line with our telephone service, and our phone would ring one long ring and two short rings for an incoming call for us. We would then pick it up and so would all the other neighbours who would listen in to catch the latest news in the community. This practice was called rubbernecking and everyone was guilty of it. There was great excitement in our house the year the transatlantic telephone cable was laid and Mom was able to call home to Germany. We could talk to our grandparents, or at least hear their voices, but the calls were terribly expensive and had to be kept short. To get around the horrendous phone bills, Mom took to using a cassette deck to record her voice and ours and would mail this to her parents. They would then answer and mail the tape back. Originally Granny ran the community's post office out of her house and the neighbours would stop in to pick up their mail from the wonderful, cubby-hole desk in the living room. When she died, Canada Post installed two green metal community mailboxes at the end of our driveway and for years we relied on a weekly mail service to deliver our letters from a large canvas sack that sat in the back of a dusty panel truck.

During the two long months of summer holidays from school, the occasional letter, the little radio, and our old black-and-white TV were our only connection to the rest of the world. When we finally got a colour television, it was a big box of a TV but we also got a second channel and BCTV joined CBC in entertaining us. I still remember coming home from school and watching *The Flintstones*, followed by *Hawaii Five-O*. The theme song to *Hawaii Five-O* was my favourite and one that stuck in my head. Barb and I also watched *The Brady Bunch* every afternoon. Those Brady kids lived in a friendly town and they could walk to their school. I really envied them. Barb and I lived in the sticks on a gravel road that was either dusty or icy, depending on the season, and we had to ride the school bus for an hour each way.

I had many reasons to hate that hour-long bus ride. I started grade 2 in 1969 at 150 Mile House where the student population was almost exclusively Indigenous children from the nearby St. Joseph's Mission. I couldn't play with the Indigenous kids; they wouldn't talk to me. They spoke their own Carrier, Shuswap and Chilcotin languages in furtive whispers at recess and lunch among each other because those languages were forbidden at the mission where they lived. I was too young to understand the global tensions I had been living among in Europe and I missed my familiar German neighbourhood. I was also too young to understand the racial tensions of rural Canada in the sixties. My grade 2 teacher very quickly moved me into the grade 3 side of her split classroom and, honestly, being a bright student didn't help matters at all when it came to me finding new friends among my classmates. There is an old photo of me from those years, an old school photo of my grade 2–3 class in 1969–1970. There I am, in the third of four rows, huddled in beside the teacher as if I am trying to disappear. The entire class, with the exception of four white faces, is brown. My bright red German hair ribbons on yellow blonde braids stand out like exclamation points. No wonder I couldn't fit in!

My pronounced "German-ness" was never more visible than when I wore hair ribbons in my braids. The other girls on the school bus were unmerciful. I remember one day, early in my first year there—it was autumn, and the leaves were falling off the golden aspens that grow everywhere in the Cariboo—when one of my schoolmates confronted me on the bus.

"Why do you wear hair ribbons?" she asked.

"Because German girls wear hair ribbons!"

"Do they wear diapers to school too?"

That last comment would have been the most stinging thing one seven-year-old could say to another back then, but I refused to show any humiliation. Instead, I insisted the German way was better, hair ribbons and all. Then I beat the offender at a spelling test. When the teacher praised me in front of the whole class, I felt vindicated; smarter and "better" than the girls who teased me.

But for all my show of "head-held-high" toughness and smarts, I remained easily bullied. I was two years younger than everyone else in my grade after grade 2. Although I was as tall as most of my classmates, I was skinny. Wearing hair ribbons and "weird" clothing from Germany didn't help either, I suppose. I must have looked like quite the easy target.

My German-ness was made stronger thanks to occasional, treasured visits to Lichtental, a suburb of Baden-Baden, where my grandparents still lived. Barb and I could keep up our German language skills as we spoke German daily. We spoke with bus drivers, the nuns in the neighbouring convent, and storekeepers, but, most of all, we listened. Whenever the Canadians from the nearby air force base flew over the city and broke the sound barrier, the windows in the houses and apartment blocks below would shake from the shock waves of the sonic boom and Omi, thinking nobody saw her, would shake her fist at the sky and say "verdammte Kanadier" (damned Canadians). Omi didn't know we were listening!

I loved Omi; more than her fist-shaking, I remember her green thumb. She had planters full of warm, spicy-smelling red geraniums all along her balcony railing on the apartment house. The bright red flowers against the sunny, beige walls of the building looked amazing from the street below. Omi and Opa's small apartment on the second of three floors in the apartment house looked like a castle to me. Unlike the ranch house to which I was now accustomed, their home had central heating and hot running water. Omi let me water her geraniums and I loved the rich smell of the flowers and the cool, tinny smell of the water. One day when I was watering her geraniums, a chimney sweep was working on the apartment house across the street. He waved to me and I was so happy because, according to German folklore, when a chimney sweep waves to you you'll have good luck. Indeed, in hindsight, the chimney sweep's blessing lasted many years. It wasn't until I reached adulthood that I started to really notice my body didn't do some things as easily as other people's bodies seemed to do.

Back home again, at twelve years old, I spent most of my time delighting in being able to do whatever I wanted and being unimpressed when I had to do what I was told. We had a series of milk cows on the ranch and I hated having to milk the cow. Dad used to milk Milly, the first milk cow, on one side of the bag while her calf sucked on the other side. Milly was out all day on Rose Hill behind the house while her calf was locked in the main corral and she was glad to come in at night to see her calf and have her bag emptied. That tradition carried on with our next milk cow, Milly's replacement. Barb named her Jenny. It was an obvious reaction to my own habit of naming our animals after the Greek gods and goddesses I was enthralled with. After Cassiopeia and Andromeda, Dad decided that Barb should have a turn naming our animals as they arrived and, hence, there was Jenny. Jenny was patient but I was not good at milking. I particularly disliked the strong smell of the cow's udder and the harsh disinfecting smell of the sudsy water I had to wash her teats with.

What I did like, however, was skipping down the hillside with a brimming bucket of milk afterwards. I could swing the bucket around in a full circle without spilling a drop of the milk. I remember my arm going up in front of me and swinging down behind me with the heavy, full bucket at the end of it and the feeling of victory in that warm, soft, fresh summer air.

I remember that feeling particularly well because at that time I was already having dreams of me unable to walk. A recurring vision of myself, stumbling onto my knees and unable to get up again, haunted my nights and occasionally even broke through my daydreams.

Dreams and even daydreams like this one continued as I got older, but they didn't seem to have any effect in my real life. One of the first times that I became aware that my body was in fact weaker than other kids' bodies was in the early 1970s when skiing started becoming popular. Until then, skiing was a European pastime but it was starting to catch on in the Cariboo.

When I was just an infant, my mother and father had gone downhill skiing in Europe on their wooden skis with the leather-strap bindings. On my ninth birthday, my parents gave me a pair of skis of my very own. We did not go to any formal ski resort like the kind my parents must have skied in Europe. Instead, I learned to ski on top of three feet of loose, dry snow in the foothills of the Cariboo Mountains. There were plenty of hills nearby. In fact, our ranch house sat at the bottom of hills on a little flat area. It was still a lot of work to ski there. I had to walk up the hill of my choice, strap on my skis and then ski down, making my own trail through the loose powder. I did that once or twice before I realized that the effort of ploughing through waist-deep snow was about the same whether I was going uphill on foot or downhill on my little skis.

A year later, when I was in grade 7, the school district started a ski program for kids and I got to go. My enthusiasm for the sport didn't grow very much, however. My classmates and I would all pile on the bus at the school one day a week for a month or two and drive to the little ski hill located just north of Williams Lake, Little Squaw Valley, and spend a few hours skiing. That little hill seemed so huge to me the first morning I got off the bus when I stared up at "The Face" run, and so extremely intimidating. It closed after some years but not before my future husband took me in hand over fifteen years later and showed me how to conquer "The Face."

Unfortunately, I accidentally misrepresented my ability on the very first day there in 1973. The teachers divided us up into groups: those who had never been on skis and those who had. I said I had been on skis; I had a pair at home. It didn't occur to me that the ski hill's rental skis came with real ski boots and step-in bindings and that the skiing there was totally different than what I had done on the ranch. I missed the first day's lessons because I was going up the rope tow with the "advanced" skiers and sliding back down the hill backwards whenever I let go of the rope. Someone eventually noticed me and I was back in the group with the beginners the next day.

I never did learn to ski through the elementary school program. I did learn other things, however. In particular, I learned how to navigate a multicultural world and how to be tough. In 1974, I started high school in grade 8 in Williams Lake. I was only eleven years old and once more without a friend. My friend Mary Anne and her family had moved to Vancouver during the summer and I missed her terribly. Nevertheless, high school proved to be a much more positive experience for me. While I had been a minority member in elementary school as one of a few white faces in a sea of brown ones, in high school there weren't many Indigenous children at all, and I had an easier time fitting in. I finally learned to keep my mouth shut. My rebellious streak seemed to mature at this time but I learned to stay silent in class and to be less competitive when it came to schoolwork. I made friends. A big wooden school desk was set in my bedroom at home for me when my grade 8 social studies teacher suggested I should have a desk to do homework at. Actually, he suggested I should start doing homework. It was a great old desk with a funny, musty smell but I did spend hours at it, doing everything and anything but homework. I wrote stories and poems, drew pictures, fantasized and daydreamed. A lot of the pictures I drew were of horses. Horses were still a major part of my life.

Grade 8 was the year when I got my own horse. I was fascinated with the creatures and I read everything about them that I could get my hands on. I knew all the breeds and colours, the "socks" and the face markings, and so it was with great pride that I accurately described my own horse one spring morning. I stood in my grade 8 home economics class and I enthusiastically told my few, new friends, "My new horse is an eight-year-old Quarter Horse and Morgan cross. She's dark brown and has a sorrel mane and tail."

"An eight-year-old Quarter Horse and Morgan cross, dark brown with a sorrel mane and tail," someone mimicked loudly across the room in a high, thin voice. "Ooh, how special." Until that moment I didn't realize how quickly you can be judged a show-off, even when you don't mean to be showing off. I was just excited.

Lucky entered my life within the next few days. She was shorter than the old ranch horse, Rebel, that I'd been riding and she was stocky, with the square shoulders and haunches of the Morgan Horse. I loved her from the start. Often too lazy to put the saddle on her, I would jump on her back and with just the bridle on her head we would simply go for a ride for the afternoon. Lucky was portly though, well-built and sturdy—OK, she was a bit fat—and my legs, although long enough to encircle her girth, were too weak to hold me in place when she started to trot. In a hurry to get back to the barn, she would jog and I would bounce, gripping her tough, wiry mane in desperation.

During that first summer between grades 8 and 9, bouncing back through the hayfield over the stubble of the cut grass one hot August afternoon, my legs succumbed to fatigue and I bounced right off Lucky's back. I don't know who was more surprised, her or me, when I ended up flat on my back in the golden stubble, winded and confused. Lucky actually stopped dead and turned her head around to regard me with, I swear, a surprised look in her eyes. After that incident, I always used a saddle and rammed my worn cowboy boots well forward in the stirrups to keep my legs and feet in place on her broad back and sides.

Hot summer afternoons were pleasantly cool in the bush and we would meander along thin paths made by the deer under the ragged bark of giant fir trees. I remember Lucky's hooves clopping gently on the hard-packed, thin soil of the path. The heavy, warm smells of the hot evergreen branches mingled with those of delicate wildflowers and accompanied us for hours. One of my favourite rides was to Wiggins Creek, kilometres from the ranch. I liked that ride the most because three-quarters of the way to the creek an old birch tree had fallen across the narrow path and its peeling trunk lay too high for Lucky to step over. The first time we came on this obstacle I learned to my delight that Lucky liked to jump. It was more of a hop, really, from a standing start but I lived for that brief moment of flight and took the path to Wiggins Creek many times solely for the purpose of flying over that jump.

The delight in that sensation of flight stayed with me, always accompanied by the smell of warm horsehair and the feel of coarse, wiry mane clenched in my fingers. Later, much later when Lucky was gone and I was riding in the woods behind a different ranch on a different horse, I would always search vainly for a log to jump over.

My high school years passed quickly and, it seems to me now, rather joyfully. I spent my days reading, writing poetry, riding Lucky through the heavily scented woods in summer and skiing around the ranch in winter. Those days of skiing were the only downside of ranch life for me, then, although I had more success with cross-country skiing than I ever did with downhill skiing. Cross-country skiing didn't involve so many hills and I was much more comfortable with it. Plus, I got real skis and boots that fit me. I must have spent some 4-H money to get the equipment because I remember the salesperson in town selling me fibreglass skis and showing me how they could bend without breaking. He informed me that if I ever ran into a tree the skis would run right up the trunk. Although he was laughing when he told me this, he wouldn't have found it funny, I'm sure, if he'd known I would put that theory to practice. I skied in the woods behind the ranch and more than once found myself going too fast on an icy cow trail and being thankful for the skis' flexibility.

Mom had her own pair of skis and she and I would also ski around the hayfield together. I didn't enjoy those outings as much as she did but I did love the sun sparking diamonds off the fresh snow. I especially loved it when the sky was that deep lovely blue and the whole world shone like a jewel. I was still a klutz and fell way more than a person should, but at least the skiing was on the level more often than not. When I skied with other people, Mom's friends and our older neighbours, I was always the last one finished, the last one to come in, though I worked at least as hard as everyone else. I could never figure that out and thought it was totally unfair.

In hindsight, which is pretty clear, it seems I've had multiple sclerosis and the resulting weakness in my legs for a long, long time.

That weakness always warred with an incredible stubbornness. I loved to move my body and the faster, the better. Naturally then, I joined the high school track and field team. I ran the sprints, the 100- and 200-metre races, and I threw the javelin. I was my own worst enemy though, thanks to my stubbornness. Two years younger than all my

41

friends, who were also on the track team, I wanted to race with them and not with my own age group when we went to track meets. Invariably, I came in close to last in the races. The one day I won my race is still a shining memory for me.

Track season was in the spring and once it was over, my love of nature was rewarded when the flower garden in the front yard of the ranch house bloomed. In grade 11, I decided I wanted a flowerbed of my own. Mom always had terrific flowerbeds in front of our house and she gave me my own spot in the front yard. I dug up a flowerbed and patiently planted bulbs. The blue grape muscari were the first to come up in the spring, in May. They were followed later in the summer by other flowers that I can't remember now but which were all planted from seed from Mom's other flowers. There were red lychees too, or Maltese Cross, maybe even a deep red tulip or a cheery daffodil or two. There were also bright blue forget-me-nots and small, white lily-of-the-valley that were formed into a corsage for me for my high school graduation.

I graduated from Columneetza High School in Williams Lake in 1979 at sixteen years old near the top of the class. My class was so large there are two grad photos. I'm sitting in the centre of one, in the very front row in a long, light blue dress. I still have the same expression on my face that I had when I was in grade 3: shoulders slightly hunched, chin forward, awkwardly shy but determined, fully confident in my ability to handle whatever was coming next.

MARRIAGE AND MOTHERHOOD

Gladly I surrender myself to love and parentage.
—Will Durant

Because I graduated early and my mother didn't think it was a good idea for me to go to university as a sixteen-year-old, I went off to Germany for six months in 1979. I lived with my aunt and uncle in the village of Weisenheim am Berg and spent my time as a foreign guest student in a German high school. I had a great time. I even learned to do ballroom dancing through an extra-curricular course in a nearby city. I remember the dark studio and the plump, blonde woman who gave us such clear instructions. I also remember my partner's initial hesitations and my own clumsy attempts at moving my feet in time to the rhythm of the music. When we were able to move together through the intricacies of polka, waltz and foxtrot, I gloried in being a member of a smoothly moving machine on the polished, dark floor. After those rather unsatisfactory adventures in skiing, it felt marvellous to be able to dance. The music soaked into my skull and took over my body. That was 1979. Now it's 2017 and I still love to feel the heavy beat of a bass drum become my heartbeat. My legs are too slow and heavy now to move in rhythm but my arms and hands seem to sway on their own and my upper body moves easily and instinctively to any music.

After my stint in Germany in 1979, I spent a summer working in the Williams Lake Visitor's Centre. I'm told that a good-looking young man came in one day with a rather ridiculous question about fishing in nearby Lac La Hache and that he was really just checking me out. The name Tom Redl didn't mean anything to me at the time, however, and I took little notice of him. I couldn't have known then about the role he would later play in my life. It would be many years until we met again and I found the reason that would keep me forever connected to the Cariboo and the ranch life I had grown up in.

At first, however, I imagined I would leave the ranch life far behind. My time spent in Europe combined with the adventures I discovered through the books I continued to read voraciously led me to dream of becoming a translator working for the UN. I dreamt of being an international career woman. I dreamt of living in cities more glamorous than the one populated by the Brady Bunch kids I had envied as a child. I started by moving to Victoria, BC, to study languages. I loved the city and the Pacific Ocean, which lay right beside the university campus, and drew me to its shores almost every day. On grey winter days, the heavy ocean swells and the tangy, salty air reminded me of how far I was from the crisp, dry air of the Cariboo. On bright spring days, the ocean tossed white wavelets against the rocks on the shorelines and I drank in the unfamiliar sights and smells, while wishing I could somehow capture this atmosphere and take it home with me. Instead of thick, quiet woods and hot, arid grasslands, here were majestic oaks, towering stone cathedrals and busy sidewalks in a bustling downtown. Catching a bus and going downtown to shop in a mall, or in Chinatown, was an adventure and I loved my feelings of freedom, independence and, most of all, competence. I also loved my courses at the University of Victoria. I still joke today that I didn't learn English until I studied German. Of course, I remember my grade 5 teacher trying to hammer English grammar into me—nouns and verbs, adjectives and adverbs—but I didn't know about the nominative, accusative and genitive cases or direct and indirect sentence objects until I started studying German in university. I added Russian for good measure. I always relied on my intuitive knowledge to guide me through English and German, but I had to really learn grammar to master Russian. With those three languages behind me, French, Italian and Spanish were easy to add to my roster of languages.

Although those years were largely spent devoting myself to my education, it was not a time of purely intellectual activity. Whenever I came home on holidays my life was full again with physical activity. My father had realized I'd grown up and could actually help out with the ranch chores. I have a vivid memory from one Christmas holiday when I was feeding the cows for Dad. I was walking along the skinny little path the cows had made to the watering hole and I fell off the path into the snow. I had been carrying an axe to chop a hole through the ice so the cows could get to the water and the axe suddenly disappeared under the soft snow, pulling my arm down with it. I clenched my muscles, hoisted the axe back onto the path and laid it there while I floundered around, trying to pull myself back up onto the path. It felt like trying to flop onto a life raft. The whole time, my feet never touched bottom. The path of packed snow, the cow trail, was like a skinny plank over the sea of loose powder snow that covered the hayfield. It was terrifying, and at the same time, it was hilarious. I was so glad nobody saw me floundering around with my face in the snow. I had known that watering hole all my life. It was the little pond where Barb and I had skated as children. The nearby hayfield was the one that Mom and I used to ski around. The familiar landscape was transformed for me that day and suddenly gave the first hints at how harsh and unforgiving it is in the Cariboo in winter. For the first time, I paid real attention to the stark beauty of the land and its demands on the minds and bodies of those who make it home. Cold snow melted and ran down my back and chest under my thick sweater and I made it back from the watering hole that day looking like I had been caught in a snowstorm, laughing at myself.

Twenty-two years later, when Tom and I were building our new house, I once again fell into loose powder snow while carrying a load of tools. This time, however, my legs were too weak to allow me to stand up. Luckily, I was within a hundred metres from our front door so I crawled through the metre-deep snow to our front step. I was able to pull myself up on the door handle and stagger into the house where I found a chair and sat until I was strong enough to brush the snow off me. Once again, I was covered head to foot with cold snow. Once again, nobody was around to witness my plight. This time though, I was angry. I was angry at myself for falling and equally angry at life for saddling me with this disease. MS has robbed me of the sense of humour I had as a young woman. When I fall, I can't laugh at myself anymore.

During my university years I returned to Miocene not only during the winter holidays but also during summer breaks. My parents had scrimped and saved enough to cover my first year's tuition and lodging expenses, but I paid for the rest of my education with summer jobs. I spent time working at the tourist centre but I also spent two summers with a better-paying but riskier job with the Ministry of Forests. I sprayed so-called noxious weeds with a deadly herbicide. Looking back now, I regret that I had next-to-no protection from the lethal spray. I was once doused thoroughly by my partner who in error nailed my head and shoulders with a jet of herbicide from one of our poison-filled tanks. If that stuff, Tordon, was already banned in the US for being lethally dangerous to people and it killed every broad-leafed plant that it touched, what do you suppose it might have done to the brain of a susceptible, young, still-growing person? My guess is it simply added to a toxic burden I was carrying and the only surprise now is that I developed multiple sclerosis later, instead of cancer.

In any case, I ended four glorious years of university study with very little student debt and a great thirst for adventure. In 1984, I graduated with a double-major bachelor of arts degree in German and Russian languages.

The minimal amount of debt I had had been incurred when I went to Russia one summer instead of staying home to work. I came back to Williams Lake in 1984 after my studies ended. I thought I was making a stopover before going off into the world to discover my destiny as a glamorous international translator but, somehow, I fell head-over-heels in love with Tom Redl. Tom turned out to be a neighbouring rancher on Horsefly Road. I gave up my idea of becoming a translator at the UN, and settled instead into a life much like the one I thought I had left behind when I departed from Miocene for Victoria four years earlier.

I knew Tom was "the one" on our first date. We went to a cowboy cabaret with another couple who were friends of mine. Tom not only got on famously with my friends, which the shy introvert in me admired tremendously, but he could dance! The first time we danced together, my body moved instinctively and effortlessly in time with his, and I loved the feel of his arms around me. Tom worked hard in the woods in those days, and it was physically demanding work. The work paid off in a strength in his arms and hands that had me in love with him after just one dance. Plus, he enjoyed dancing as much as I did! I felt sure we would stay happy together.

On June 27, 1987, Tom and I were married in a big family wedding ceremony in the United Church in Williams Lake. Our reception was at the community club hall in Miocene. In June, all the native flowers are in bloom in the Cariboo and I never see the pink wild roses, blue lupins, and red paintbrush now without being reminded of our wedding day. Our first son, Ben, was born in 1988, followed by Sam in 1990 and our daughter Lexie (Alexandra) in 1992. Marriage and the swiftly following motherhood meant a return to the isolation of ranch life in the Cariboo. Tom and I moved onto his parents' ranch and I slowly but surely lost touch with my social group from university. Although the lifestyle was, in its own way, rather lonely, I also thought it was romantic to live in the back-of-beyond with nobody around me but my husband and my immediate family. It was a return to my childhood roots, but this time I was in charge and I flourished. Like any good young ranch woman, I had a lot of energy and raising three children wasn't enough work for me. One of the first things I tried to set up at our new house on the ranch was a garden. I did it the old pioneer way with a shovel, a rake, and a hoe. I remember clearly the spade edge slicing through the green, root-filled sod, and then leaning on the spade to flip up the square of grass and weeds I had just outlined and turning the sod over to reveal pale, stony, dry and dusty soil underneath. My wonderful father-in-law Ed drove out the loader machine with buckets full of well-rotted manure from the ranch's silo area and dumped it in our little garden, which Tom had fenced off with expensive page wire. The September when I first pulled huge fat potatoes out of their hidden places in the garden, I turned them over in my hands with a grin that stretched across my face. I felt like I was part of a Thanksgiving church service.

My connection with nature was not limited to my gardening. I also loved the songbirds, especially during spring and fall when they were most plentiful, filling the air with their melodies. The black and yellow evening grosbeaks came to our bird feeders regularly and, together with the red-winged blackbirds, they went through the sunflower seeds I put out for them at a tremendous rate. There were sometimes over forty of these bigger birds in the aspen trees outside the dining room window, joined by smaller birds like red-capped house finches, grey chickadees and brown sparrows. Sometimes I'd see a big, brown northern flicker join the throng, perching on top of the feeder to reach the suet hung high above it. Of course, there was also the Boeing 747 of the bird world: the pileated woodpecker. He would perch on our roof and try to drill into the metal TV antenna every morning at dawn. Him, I didn't enjoy so much.

More than birds, it was horses that I adored. They remained one of the most beloved aspects of ranch life for me. I simply worshipped those animals. Once married and with children, I still continued to ride whenever I could. It was in the mid-nineties when I bought another horse. Corky was a red-brown mare—a bonafide bay with black mane and tail. She also came with an attitude. I continued to have my old trouble with generalized weakness in my legs and that made gripping my new horse's sides tightly nearly impossible. She quickly learned to take advantage of that and would try to go wherever she wanted, ignoring the demands of the bit in her mouth. It was a contest of wills, which I often lost. However, Corky and I would occasionally reach a compromise that suited us both, like on one particular warm May afternoon shortly after I had bought her. We were in a newly ploughed field and the air was so thick and soft with the smell of fresh soil and grass that I felt like I could float on it. Corky wanted to run and I let her. Suddenly, I was flying, like I had that first day so long ago with Grampa's white Blanco. I was buoyed along on that wonderful air with a tangled mane once again grasped tightly in my fist. I was incredibly happy with my ranch life that day.

Other rides on Corky were for business only but I still enjoyed them and found comfort in the "eye candy" nature provided in the thick woods behind the ranch. Every spring we turned the cattle out on range. They needed to be pushed along from our ranch through a neighbouring ranch, up a hill and finally through a gully to get out to our summer range. Two hundred cows with their calves make a lot of noise and dust and it was always a long day, even on a horse. Corky actually lost her temper with the slow pace of the herd one memorable day and, in exasperation, reached out and bit the slow-moving cow in front of her on the rump. I shared her exasperation and patted her neck in approval.

The best part of those rides was the ride home. Free of the traffic jam of ponderously moving bovines and eager to get home and get the load—me—off her back, Corky would pick up her feet and run home. She had a beautiful, smooth lope and the wind would lift my hair off my hot neck and dry the sweat on my back through my thin shirt.

One day on the ride back I saw the valley beside me covered in a dusty, yellow haze that clung thickly to the evergreens on the opposing hillside. I wondered out loud what it was.

"Pollen," one of the older ranchers riding with us told me. "The trees are pollinating now. It will be a good crop of cones later this year by the looks of it."

Moments like that have turned into memories that stay with me. The dark green conifers dusted with a fine, yellow powder under a thick, yellowish haze were so visual and sensual that it shook my confidence in myself as a native of the area. I hadn't ever seen this before. The surprise was both unsettling and uplifting. I was witnessing resilience in nature and the process of regeneration as well as nature's stubborn determination to carry on.

Unfortunately, the ranch's natural beauty was not always enough to keep me from wondering about the life I'd given up by staying on the land. Life in busy, populated Germany and then in beautiful, bustling Victoria was a welcome change from an isolated ranch for childhood and a poor preparation for an isolated ranch as a young mother. The independent, modern woman of the world I had envisioned becoming had disappeared. Although I loved being a wife and mother, there were times when I battled depression and wondered about the dreams I had entertained while in university. As a rancher, I had less time for my precious books, papers, and foreign languages and had to devote more time to getting down and dirty with nature: haying, calving, shovelling snow, gardening, swatting mosquitoes, and still more snow-shovelling. I loved so much of my rural life but I also ached for something to do that was mine alone, something I could do that would contribute not only to my family and small Cariboo community but to society at large. Eventually, I settled on writing. It was a good fit: I had always been capable with language, I have always had a vivid imagination and wild creativity, and writing was something I could do from home without driving to town and fretting about leaving my children for hours without me in a strange daycare facility. Both they and I were used to having each other always present in our lives.

One of my first exploits was to go to the tiny Williams Lake library and look up local authors. It didn't take long to find Ann Walsh's works. Here was a well-known author who actually lived in Williams Lake! I wanted to be a famous writer like she was but I didn't have the nerve to look her up in the telephone book and give her a call to get some advice. Instead, I signed out a couple of her books and took them home to study her craft. It was the beginning of my journey as a writer and it gave me the balance I needed with my commitment to my family and our ranching life and my desire to communicate with the bigger world.

Time for reading and writing, and time for pleasure-riding with Corky, was clawed out of a frenetic schedule of chores in those days. It could be overwhelming to look after three children, support Tom with the ranch work, and find time to celebrate with our extended family. The women of the family took turns hosting the Christmas dinner. One year when it was my turn I had a two-year-old and a six-month-old and a baby on the way when I prepared a sit-down, multi-course Christmas dinner for twenty-three in our tiny log house. I fretted about hosting that dinner for a year, from Boxing Day the previous year when I knew it was my turn. When the time came, although it was a massive amount of work for me, I pulled it off. Looking back now, I shake my head both at how I had the energy to complete that challenge and at how naive I was to think I had to put myself through that. A more confident and older me would have flat-out refused the burden.

I was usually lucky with the family around us though. Although the ranch was isolated in many ways and friends were few and far between, Tom and I were surrounded by both his family and mine, and that meant our children grew up with loving grandparents always available to help out with whatever was needed. Eventually, too, Horsefly Road was paved, and that made the effort of going into town less of a challenge than it was in my childhood. Our kids got the benefit of playschool and friends outside of their own siblings. For the most part, however, our kids had a true ranch childhood like the one I'd enjoyed. My mother still tells the story of the time when Ben, my eldest child, was little and we had all walked up

Rose Hill on a hot, sunny afternoon in the strong summer heat. We picked saskatoons from the big bush and then we sat down and looked at the view. From up there you can see Beaux Yeux Lake. Ben, who was just in school then, told Mom exactly how he would run irrigation lines across the hill, pumping water from that lake. He had it all figured out.

A few years later, one of his teachers approached me with a worried face and said, "Do you know that Ben walks back and forth in the playground at lunch, in short, repeated segments, talking to himself?"

I laughed. "He's moving imaginary irrigation lines."

In 1991 Tom and I moved out of his tiny log cabin and built a house on the property we purchased next door to the ranch. Our love of the outdoors meant we put big windows in our house, so as much of the outside could come in as possible. I spent as much time as I could outside. In the summers, I would often be found on a tractor in the hayfield in the hot sun, a toddler perched beside me and the tall grass falling into fresh windrows beside the tractor as I cut hay. Or I would be in the silage truck, with a toddler still beside me, roaring down a dusty, bumpy ranch road to bring the cut hay from the silage machine in the field up to the silo for storage. Or finally I was in the silage machine, guiding it along the sweet-smelling, freshly cut windrows it gobbled up and dumping its load of chopped hay into the truck that then shuttled it up to the silo. Work as a ranch hand was considered by all to be vital then and we finally began coping with the demands of children by hiring babysitters, thus freeing me up to work in the fields.

It didn't occur to me then that the workload was tremendous and maybe too much for me to handle. Cooking, cleaning house, raising children and haying were jobs that consumed twenty hours of a day. One day it really was too much. It was 1999, high summer, and the middle of haying season on the ranch. I found myself sitting on the ground in the hayfield beside the silage chopper, unable to drive it anymore. When Tom came running over and found me unable even to speak, he firmly ordered me back to the house. I took a week off from ranch work, then, and drove my young children to Kamloops for a mini-holiday for the four of us. It was in Kamloops that my right side went numb, from my spine right around my torso to my breastbone.

The strange numbness lasted six weeks. I found out years later that it was an early symptom of full-blown MS. At the time I dismissed it as overwork and stress.

That mini Kamloops holiday—or desperate respite, which is how I look at it now—was not the only vacation I took with the kids during my years of being a young mother. Both Tom and I like to travel. Early in our married life we couldn't afford to do a lot with the limited time and money we had, but we still had some memorable trips. At first

Tom's parents, Trudy and Ed, lent us their camper and truck for our little holidays. The first year we were married and Ben was only about six months old, we borrowed the "rig" and drove to Vancouver Island and did some camping and sightseeing there and on Salt Spring Island as well. The second trip happened when Ben wasn't quite two. We drove down to Nakusp and through the Kootenays and southern BC. Then Trudy and Ed gave us their old camper when they bought a fifth wheel (in return we bought them a motor for their small fishing boat). The camper was decorated seventies style, with brown and beige seat cushions, orange curtains and a beige-brown shag carpet on the floor that revealed an orangey-brown linoleum in mint condition when we pulled it up to sell the camper in our turn, years later.

We mounted that camper on the back of an old Ford truck we bought for $800. I named it the Blue Moose, because the hood and the doors were different shades of blue, and with the orange and brown camper mounted on the back, we looked like the Beverly Hillbillies when we took it out for an outing. The holidays we did in the Blue Moose were driving holidays. One was when Ben was about eight, Sam six and Lexie four. We all piled in and drove to Jasper, then down the Icefields Parkway to Banff, through the Rockies to Castlegar and Cranbrook and home again via the Kootenays and Kamloops. It was a great trip, and we camped along the way in our Blue Moose. I still tell the story of the time the Blue Moose almost got a speeding ticket. The old truck could barely reach the speed limit as it trundled down the highway but one time, when Tom had managed to get the beast actually going the speed limit, we missed the speed reduction sign just outside of Fernie. The young policeman who pulled us over could barely contain his grin when he looked in the back seat and saw the three little children. He finally settled for a "written warning" and a bent-over, belly-holding roar of laughter.

The children were slowly growing older, less needy and definitely more independent as they worked their way through school. When they were at elementary school, the same school I had attended at the 150, I spent a lot of time there volunteering and I got to know the teachers and students quite well. I was the parent who read with the classroom, taught students a bit of French and helped them with their computer work. I was also the parent who sat on the hillside to watch the school's track and field day every year and the parent who was bursting with pride as Lexie won race after race.

Watching Lexie run brought back memories of my high school days and the track team. I remembered the feeling of running, with the air brushing my skin as I moved and my ponytail bouncing behind me, and I missed those days. By then, in 2002, I was already all too aware of a weakness in my body and I blamed it on having had three children in five years. I was slightly overweight and so, in the spring of 2002, I decided impulsively to join a road-running group in Williams Lake. Surely, I thought, I could run this weight off and "muscle up" my legs. Tom cared for the kids when I went to town to run and I made some new friends with the running group. One day, one of my new friends ran up behind me and said, "Do you know that your left foot hits the ground flatter than your right foot? Your gait is off." I quickly blamed my running shoes, the weather and anything else I could think of but not my body itself. Shortly afterwards, I sprained my left ankle. Again, I was quick to dismiss it, blaming a bump in the road or my shoes.

Hindsight really is twenty-twenty. My gait was off and my left leg was moving differently than the right due to the MS that was making its presence known in my body. I just didn't want to deal with that yet.

The instinct I had on that long-ago first date with Tom, that he was the one, continued to ring true. Our marriage is a happy one. One thing I always appreciated about Tom was his willingness to take time out to spend with his family. Vacations were important family time and now with the children all in school we had to fit vacations into a small slot in late June, between classrooms and haying season. Nevertheless, we managed to see a lot of the country with the kids.

One holiday with the children was to the badlands in Alberta, to the fabulous dinosaur exhibit in Drumheller.

We took shorter trips too, week-long vacation drives, and we still talk about all those trips—but especially the six-week-long cross-Canada one where we pulled the kids out of school early and on which, for some reason, the kids decided they had to see the legislative buildings in each province and territory. We missed only Nunavut's and that is now on every bucket list in the family. The summer we did that trip across Canada became a turning point for me. With my ankle still wrapped in a supportive bandage in late June 2002, I piled into our truck with Tom, Ben, Sam and Lexie and we headed out to see our country. Crossing Canada in our truck and Ed's borrowed fifth-wheel trailer for me meant marvelling again at the beauty and diversity of this country, from the Rockies to the red sands of PEI. I'd seen the red sands of PEI once before, when as a teenager I went on a sponsored trip, but I marvelled at them just as much as I did any of the new sights. It was amazing to surround myself with such diverse landscapes before coming home to resume ranch chores and start another haying season. I had plenty to see and think about, so I shouldn't have spent any time worrying about my walking gait, but a feeling of heaviness and despondency was always there in the back of my mind, weighing me down.

Slowly I was forced to start paying attention to my body and what it was trying to tell me. I began to really notice exhaustion while I was director of the Pacific National Exhibition (PNE) when the children were making the transitions to high school. By then, they were a little older and were spending more time away from home on trips of their own, and with more time on my hands I jumped at the chance to become involved in affairs outside the ranch. I enjoyed those years working the PNE; the children were still young enough to be thrilled by the opportunities offered by the PNE's Playland and the fair in general, and I liked being more involved in life outside my little community. More and more, however, for some reason I couldn't fathom, my duties as a public face of the fair exhausted me and I found it hard to maintain a cheerful persona. The exhaustion never left me, in fact, and it merely intensified as each fair season rolled around. I finally resigned when I realized that I wasn't recovering from my monthly trips to board meetings in time to be a good mother and help with my family's activities. Hindsight is crystal clear, isn't it? Overwhelming fatigue is another one of the first symptoms of MS.

Fatigue is, however, also the first symptom of many a disease. I dragged myself into my doctor's office, complaining about the fatigue. Finally, my doctor ordered a blood test and that test showed that I was suffering from hypothyroidism. In other words, an under-functioning thyroid gland. That diagnosis stunned me. I knew I was more tired than I should be, but I also knew that as a mother with three children I had every right to be tired. I still remember grumbling about having to take thyroid pills every day, knowing that I would be taking them for the rest of my life. I also have a hazy memory of reading about hypothyroidism and the Cassandra-like warning that it was often connected to more serious diseases like multiple sclerosis. I had no time in my life for a serious disease or even an inconvenient one like hypothyroidism. I was simply too busy with my life and work on our ranch and my children. Although the children were becoming more independent, they still took up a lot of time and I wanted to be there for all of it. I still like to joke that as the children grew I traded in washing diapers for driving. I drove those kids everywhere: science fairs, track meets, 4-H meetings, birthday parties, school concerts and more. My life was full. I wasn't going to let a little fatigue get in the way of doing what I wanted. In addition to staying active as a wife, mother, and ranch hand, I was becoming increasingly serious about pursuing a writing career. I often remembered that my great-grandmother Mary Sillars Mackenzie was a poet; somewhere I have a duo-tang folder of her poems that Dad found and gave to Barb to type up a long time ago. Opa was a writer of non-fiction pieces. I decided I must have talent for writing from both sides of the family. I wanted to write too. Specifically, I wanted to be like Ann Walsh. And so, as it often happens when you want something, fate conspires to make it happen.

Verena Berger called me up out of the blue one day, wanting me to edit something she had written. She knew I spoke both German and English fluently and was worried about her writing, as English is her second language. Before I knew what was happening, I had joined her and another one of her friends in a writing group. Then Ann Walsh joined us. Ann Walsh joined our writing group! I could hardly believe my luck. That writing group was invaluable to me; not only did it provide some publishing opportunities but it was the beginning of some really strong friendships. The group consisted of Verena, Ann, Donna, Anne with an "e," and me. It was a small group but somehow the five of us worked into a very productive group, and for most of us, writing turned from a hobby into a profession. We are all, now, published writers.

I got on well with Ann right away. She was excited to learn that I was a rancher and rode horses. Early on, she brought her granddaughter out to the ranch. I saddled up a horse and helped the young girl up, then climbed a corral fence and sat there, watching her ride. The worn fence rails were warm and rough in the sunshine that day and I remember while I watched the girl ride I fought down the urge to get Corky in, saddle her up and do circles in the corral too for the sheer pleasure of the ride.

Later on we had tea back in the house and Ann thrilled my children with generous gifts of her books. Her granddaughter still wore the same smile she had on the horse.

I rode Corky regularly in those days, but I was finding it more and more of a chore to get the saddle on her back, get it cinched up and then ride her with a commanding grip of my legs. The day Corky disagreed with my wish to turn left on a ranch road and reared in protest is another vivid memory. I didn't come out of the saddle, but I was shaken. The horse knew I was not in control and that is not a good feeling when you're riding a strong-willed horse. Still, I held on to the hope that things would get better and I turned Corky back out into the field with the other horses on the ranch. Looking back on those days of riding Corky brings up a strange mixture of joy and regret. I was too busy and still too healthy to dwell on the increasing signs of illness entering my life. It niggled a bit at the back of my mind that all was not well but I blamed it on the heavy load of chores and obligations that consumed my days.

The one thing that always made me feel better was my ability to let my imagination run free and create wonderful dream-worlds. Dream-worlds are handy to have on hand when you want to write and I love writing. It seems to me that my writing life is symbolized by, of all things, a rock. I have a rock on my desk here at home; it's a red, yellow, and faintly black-striped thing that almost glows. It is a little smaller than my fist and I have large hands. It is unnaturally smooth for a rock that was found outside of water. Tom found it on top of Rose Hill behind the old house where I grew up. It was a late spring day—

must have been 2002 or 2003—and we were busy putting up the new fence around the grazing lease. We'd just bought an uncle's piece of the old ranch and it was still many years before Dad signed his share of his parents' original ranch over to us. Tom picked up the rock and gave it to me. I remember walking down from that mountain-top that day with the rock in my coat pocket and the fresh, crisp smell of the pine and fir forest all around me and having a vision.

I'd been thinking of writing and wondering how my career as a writer would look and if I could make it all work. A feeling washed over me, through the trees and the air around me, like a quiet voice assuring me that everything would work out, that I would have small successes in writing, like magazine articles. I did, actually, later on. I spent four or five years writing the Open Range column for *Canadian Cowboy Country Magazine*, based on our ranch life and on memories from growing up.

I would love to have a vision like that again, to know that things are going to work out exactly the way I want them to. The first thing I was told about having MS, though, is that there are no guarantees. Nobody knows what is going to happen. Life has always managed to throw surprises my way, some bigger than others, but, in hindsight, most of them have turned out to be good surprises.

In August 2003, when the kids were solidly in their teens, Tom and I took the whole family on another holiday. This time we were going to the Arctic Ocean. We drove along the Dempster Highway to Inuvik. It was an incredible drive. Part of it felt like being on top of the world as the highway snaked along rolling mountain ridges, dropped into valleys, and took us onto a ferry to cross the Mackenzie River. Thick clouds of smoke from forest fires in Alaska rolled through the valleys below the highway and sent tendril-like arms around the mountains in the range we were following north. Inuvik itself was a rough little village and the only beautiful thing about it in my eyes was the church shaped like an igloo. We had an awesome flight over the Mackenzie Delta to Tuktoyaktuk, above the muddy braids of the Mackenzie River below us. Tuk is an Inuvialuit community. It had an otherworldly feel to it, sitting alone out on the tundra. We dipped our toes in the Arctic Ocean, toured the hamlet of Tuk, and flew back to Inuvik. Then we drove for two days again to get back to Whitehorse. From there we drove up to Dawson City and took the Top of the World highway into Alaska. That was where it all fell apart for me. I'd held it together, fighting tremendous fatigue and lethargy to cook for the family and laugh, joke and pretend everything was OK all throughout that holiday, but when we decided to climb up to the look-out on the border between Alaska and the Yukon, well, that was it.

I remember Lexie sitting at the summit of the climb, grinning and mugging for a photo with a backdrop of sharp and bare mountain peaks poking through clouds of thick, grey forest-fire smoke, and I had the camera so I managed to hold myself upright long enough to take that picture. My legs were so weak and my balance so bad that I could barely make the climb up, and coming down I was practically on my hands and knees. I ignored it. By then I was used to the invisible daily fight for strength and balance but this was the first time it was really visible to others, and Tom was alarmed.

"We're getting you to a doctor."

THE LINES ARE DRAWN

If there is no struggle, there is no progress.
—Frederick Douglass

The year after that trip to the Arctic Ocean and Alaska was an exhausting one. It was a year of doctors' visits, internists, naturopaths, and doom-prophesying, multiple sclerosis fore-warning physiotherapists until I finally found a friendly gynaecologist—of all people—who also recognized the ghastly spectre of multiple sclerosis for what it was and took action herself to set my life on the path towards a correct diagnosis. She suspected the worst when she noticed my fatigue and foot-drop during an otherwise routine visit and she left me no choice but to believe her that this was something I needed to address seriously.

"Who is your doctor?" she barked.

I reluctantly gave her a name, sure I was getting him in trouble. I was even surer when she wrote his name down on a prescription pad with a sniff of disgust and announced,

"You need to see a neurologist, stat. I'll prod this guy to send you."

When I went back to see her following the Kamloops neurologist's diagnosis of MS, she asked me gently, "How do you feel about it?"

"Relieved," I said honestly, adding, "now I have an excuse for not being able to keep up and not doing things I don't really want to do."

She laughed. "Some days," she confided, "I wish I had an excuse to bow out of things I don't want to do."

The focus of my life shifted after that trip to Kamloops in May of 2004. My entire outlook on life was disrupted, suddenly, rudely, and abruptly. Although I tried to reason that nothing had really changed—I just had a label for something that had been true for a long time—I felt like I was suddenly, immediately disabled: the victim of a chronic, incurable disease.

I read some more and started to build up a knowledge of my new disease's reality. Now that I had a name for the reason I was so tired and so weak, I wanted to know more about it. The problem was, and still is, that multiple sclerosis is a vague type of disease. That is to say, that despite decades of research, nobody knows what causes MS. You can't take a pill to make it go away. Lifestyle, environmental, genetic and biological factors all contribute to the disease, according to current evidence. I discovered

I would probably never know how or why I ended up with MS. The one straw of comfort I could find was in the fact that the disease is not "usually" fatal and people with MS can expect a normal lifespan. Unfortunately, though, people with MS experience slow but steady increases in their level of disability. This wasn't something to be cheerful about and it weighed heavily on my mind. I would probably live until I was eighty years old, but from now on as a handicapped person! I already knew extreme fatigue first-hand, lack of coordination, and generalized weakness in my legs. The more I learned about MS, the more I worried. MS symptoms could include vision problems, bladder problems, cognitive impairment and mood changes. Or not. Nobody knew what was coming for my future, least of all me. All I knew for sure was that I was in for a rough ride.

My first thought after that Kamloops trip was how to tell my family that my life, and probably theirs, had changed. I was no longer strong. I knew it would be hard for my parents but I worried, too, about my children; I was invincible in their eyes. I hated to shatter that vision. I decided to be blunt and let the children know as soon as we returned from Kamloops.

"Are you going to die?" Lexie wanted to know.

"Someday, yes. Everyone dies someday," I tried clumsily to be reassuring. "But I'm not going to die for a long time."

My mother already suspected the worst; telling my parents was merely confirming their fears. Telling my friends was a lot easier, in comparison, than talking to family. I telephoned some, emailed others.

Angela was one of the friends I told over the phone. We first met around 1994. Our daughters, both born in 1992, were the same age, and Lexie and Tamara went to preschool together. Angela and I were close. It was a difficult phone call to make, but Angela was solidly reassuring when I gave her the bad news.

"That's not what I wanted to hear," she said, and that is the only negative thing she has ever said to me about my circumstances. She has been solidly behind me, encouraging me to do things with her and very aware that my physical circumstances have changed. For example, when we go on a road-trip together now, Angela always drives. She doesn't ask, just gets in the driver's seat and is ready to go. When, in 2014, I was finally in a wheelchair, that didn't slow her down at all. She simply picked up the wheelchair and loaded it in the back of the car while I was arranging myself in the passenger seat. I know I am lucky to have her as a friend.

I know I am also lucky to have my writers' group. Back when I first got the diagnosis, the group was still a new pleasure in my life, and it wasn't until I was sitting in front of my computer, ready to email the friends in my writers' group, that my MS diagnosis really hit me. That email was different, somehow. It confirmed the horrible diagnosis in my own mind. It was my first foray into telling the world, or at least my world, about my problem, and somehow, if I told people who were still almost strangers, that would make it real. The other thing it did, that hurt me the most, was that it threatened my sense of self. I was starting to identify as a writer with this group. I was a bona fide member of the writers' group and now I was "different." It didn't feel or seem like a good difference, either. I had to carry a different label from now on: the disabled writer. I was admitting it and accepting the reality. I burst into tears. And I swear, in that moment, when I was in tears and in front of my computer screen on a grey, miserable and rainy day in June, the clouds parted and a shaft of sunshine broke through my window and bathed my computer and me in warm, golden light. A feeling washed over me, like a feeling of being hugged, and something said, "It's going to be alright. You're going to be alright."

I admit freely that in the intervening years when I've struggled with this disease, particularly when I've taken a fall and can't get up, I've looked to the sky and said, "You promised. What's with this, then?" There's never been an answer to my accusation but deep down I know that I'm heard.

After I finished telling people about my diagnosis and assured everyone that I would fight back any way I could, I attempted to draw a battle line. The line was simple. It was to stop doing things I didn't want to do anyway. I thought about my conversation with the friendly gynaecologist who admitted she sometimes wished she could get out of doing things, too. I wished it hadn't taken the diagnosis to make me realize that life was too short to waste on anything I didn't really enjoy. Although I would miss being as involved in some community events, I did not regret the great excuse I had now to get out of spending hours doing things like peeling apples and making pies for the band fundraiser at school. There were other things about ranch life I would come to miss, things like being out in the field in the early morning when the scent of a new day is just rising from the grasses, but I had to stop trying to spend hours as a ranch hand chopping hay into silage or making it into bales. I had to become more careful of my time and I had to be very careful with the limited amount of energy I now knew I had. I didn't want to spend hours listening to other people complain about their own aches and pains and how life was treating them unfairly. I wanted to spend time doing things I found important and working to stay positive. The main consideration, of course, is that I found most activities physically exhausting and I felt instinctively that I should conserve my strength. I had a limited supply of energy to get myself and my family through the day.

Most of my friends and family were supportive and encouraged me to try a new selfish lifestyle. Some of them didn't get it though. Some loved ones continued to make the same requests of me and demands on my time. I don't believe that all of them were being thoughtless. I didn't look sick—my MS symptoms weren't very visible yet— and I bet it was hard for them to accept how I felt. I imagine that most of them wanted to carry on as if everything was normal, that life was as it had always been. I wanted to carry on, too, but unlike them, I was actually living inside of my body and had much more persistent reminders that things were not the same. In truth, despite my efforts to draw and then observe my battle lines, I carried on much as I had done before. I didn't say "no" very often. A large part of my refusal to alter my lifestyle was a sense of duty and good old-fashioned pride. There is a long history for my pioneer family in our little community and I didn't want to let the community down. As much as I could, I continued to volunteer for community services and to be part of the hosting duties on the ranch.

My first year of living with the diagnosed burden of multiple sclerosis was disheartening. Because I didn't say "no" as much as I perhaps should have, I paid in fatigue, an overwhelming fatigue, which has always been the worst burden of this disease. Whenever I did say "no," though, I also felt terrible. It was a lose-lose situation. I hated that I had to rest so often. I wanted to be positive but I resented my lack of energy. I resented that I could no longer be carefree and thoughtless in giving away my time.

I resented that I felt like I had to ration out my energy. I worried I would be getting less out of life because of the rationing, but I found it increasingly necessary as my energy depleted. With the fatigue wearing me down and making me vulnerable, fear came on strongly. I worried I would become a burden to my family. I worried about the future.

Specifically, I would fret, "How bad is this thing going to get?" and "Does it end with a wheelchair, or worse?" These thoughts hit me particularly hard whenever I found myself lying down for a rest in the middle of the day.

Ranch life is very physical and can be demanding, but it was the social obligations that came my way that always seemed the most burdensome. Working in nature never tired me quite as much as did the get-togethers with neighbours or extended family members. Those get-togethers required hours of time in the kitchen peeling, slicing, and cooking. I didn't want to say "no"—or at least I didn't want to *have* to say no to such activity—but I always seemed to pay for it. I was constantly tired and grumpy. Still, a deeply ingrained stubborn streak pushed me forward. It was a steep learning curve; as time went on, I eventually became better about trusting my energy and knowing when to say "no" and when to say "yes."

But it definitely took me awhile to figure out what kind of balance I needed. For example, that first summer in 2004, the local community club desperately needed someone to cull its little library at the nearby community hall.

I volunteered for the job. One hot July Saturday, I loaded some two hundred books out of the Community Club
Library and took them to the Salvation Army. That same
day I swam fifty lengths at the pool and met a good friend
for lunch at the A&W when they were hosting a car wash
to raise funds for MS. Plus I bought a box of cherries, a
crate of blueberries and a flat of raspberries, washed and
froze the berries, and started making a German rumtopf
for Christmas. I also managed to start knitting a sweater
that evening.

Those early post-diagnosis years, I definitely took on
more labour than I needed to and often more than I wanted
to. I almost couldn't help myself. I am simply a stubborn
over-achiever. But perhaps that same stubbornness, sometimes my own enemy, is also what makes me so capable of
fighting back, of refusing to let MS take over my life.

Sometimes I wished I had the guts to say "No," or even,
"Bugger off. I'm ill." But I never did. I wasn't really angry
at the people who asked me for things; I was angry at the
disease. And the disease was not an obvious marker on me
yet, which made it more difficult for people to understand. I
really didn't look disabled then; I walked with a very slight
limp but I still walked a lot and was proactive in the community. To look at me, people would have no idea that MS was
tearing up my muscles and grinding down my strength. The
fight was invisible to all but those who knew me best.

Slowly but surely, however, people I had known for

years would stop me in the grocery store in Williams Lake to tell me how tired I looked. Some people would cross the street to avoid talking to me at all. I didn't hold it against them. I knew they didn't know what to say to me anymore. I had been so open about the diagnosis that word had spread almost instantly through my acquaintances in Williams Lake and Miocene.

The times when I felt most like my old, confident self were when I went to spend time with my writing group in Williams Lake. I drove to town once a week for Wednesday Writers' Group and I felt free to be me—Heidi.

In the summer of 2004, after the diagnosis, I finally accepted reality and I sold Corky to a good home and a very competent rider who could handle her stubbornness. I didn't look for a replacement horse. If I needed one and I could still ride, I could use a ranch hor—se. I kept my saddle, though, the one I had had since I was a child, the tooled leather saddle whose worn girth strap barely reached around Lucky's belly and cinched up so smoothly around Corky.

A few days after selling Corky, I went to town to the weekly writers' meeting at my friend Verena's house. It was a lovely summer day with a clear blue sky. It was the kind of day that would normally have me bubbling over with enthusiasm for writing, for life itself.

Ann noticed it first. "What's wrong? You're awfully quiet today."

"Nothing." I brushed the query off but she persisted until I finally grudgingly admitted that I had had to sell my horse because my legs were getting weaker and weaker.

Ann thankfully dropped the subject then and neither she nor Verena pursued it further but Ann told me years later that she went home and cried at my heartbreak and loss. She had dropped the subject, though, because she knew I didn't like talking about it. "You would have bitten my head off," she recently claimed.

It's true. I have never, ever liked talking about my problems or weaknesses. I could tell people about my diagnosis, as I felt it explained the way I now presented myself in society. It explained the way I limped and dragged my left leg when I walked. I could then be the one who took control of a conversation and focus instead on what I *was* still able to do and how I was moving through life still as a capable woman *despite* the burden of disease I was carrying. In hindsight, it was almost a case of "Look at me, look how well I'm doing with this handicap," and it was a way to keep my pride.

Losing is hard for someone who is proud. Over the years as a rancher, I had gotten used to losing animals. Animals have shorter lives than we do and they die. It always hurts though. Lucky developed crippling arthritis and couldn't move anymore shortly after I brought her to Tom's ranch. I still remember driving her into the horse sale in town, knowing she was going to go as a "meat horse," since she was unrideable anymore. I hoped that knowledge might absolve me of the guilt of avoiding having to put her down and organize a burial place on the ranch for her. I took the easy way out with Lucky and remember standing at her pen in the auction barn, ridden with that horrible guilt and looking at her soft eyes one last time. Lucky looked back, then deliberately tossed her head and turned her weary, stiff hindquarters in my direction. My tears disappeared in a sniff of a laugh and I thanked Lucky for her stubborn, independent spirit. She was not going to absolve me of this.

In contrast, when I sold Corky it was a relief. Corky was never as close to me as Lucky had been and any horse that threatens to dump its rider is untrustworthy, in my opinion. I simply didn't have the strength to deal with Corky anymore. No, what bothered me the most when I sold Corky was that I was losing the ability to ride and the combination of debilitating disease and stubborn horse had defeated me. I hated to lose, and still do.

After the loss of Corky, I continued to rely on the friendships in my writing group. Thanks to the support and mentorship of Ann and the others in the group, I continued to write over the years and slowly became a professional writer, concentrating on magazine articles and columns. In 2004 I had my first article published in *Canadian Cowboy Country*, which was followed by a regular gig as a columnist for that magazine. The airplane of my long ago dream—I AM—turned out to be a professional writer living with MS, flying above the physical ravages of the disease. In addition to writing for *Canadian Cowboy Country Magazine* for years while I was a working rancher, I also had articles published in *Macleans*, *Canadian Geographic*, many smaller American magazines, and several stories in anthologies published by Heritage House Press in BC. In 2005 I even taped a segment for CBC Radio's *OutFront* program on preg-testing on a cattle ranch. They continue to run that segment, even now, and I love to imagine the look on the businessmen's faces when they're driving to their restaurant lunch in Toronto and a herd of cows starts bawling out of their car radio. I wrote about everything: the Mad Cow devastation that hit the ranching industry, the challenges of trying to be green and recycling responsibly when living far from a recycling depot, and also, in a piece in the short-lived *Abilities Magazine,* about doing yoga with MS.

I had been diagnosed with MS, but I was determined not to give up doing the things I loved doing, especially writing and riding. Weak legs or not, I wanted to ride with the herd on turn-out day in June that second year of officially having MS.

It was 2005 and I had been without Corky for almost a year.

When I showed up at the barn with my hat in place

and my boots on, I was presented with a thin, old palomino mare from the ranch herd.

My nephew greeted me, "Take Paige, Aunt Heidi," he said. "She doesn't run or jump anymore. She'll be perfect for you."

Of course. I swallowed my disappointment and grief. What was I expecting? With an ache I remembered jumping over that fallen log with my beloved Lucky. It was hard to face the fact that the days of riding Lucky and Corky and galloping along forest paths or ducking under thick branches in pursuit of an errant cow were over and so were the days of finding solace in discovering nature's surprises in the woods: thick, green clumps of moss beside a quiet, thin black rill of water; pale pink-brown mushrooms sprouting from a rotten log; and the old scar of a pioneer's blaze on the trunk of a large tree which once marked his own trail through the woods.

I would just have to try to enjoy my ride with Paige. As promised, she was quiet. From her back, between her gracefully pointed ears, I watched the dusty road and the rumps and backs of two hundred cows and calves move ponderously along to the range. I didn't try to detour into the lovely woods, not once. Neither Paige nor I would have been able to do that. When I got home that afternoon my nephew unsaddled Paige for me. I took my saddle into the barn and hung it up beside his tack, thus giving it to him. I never rode again.

Because the support and friendship of the writers' group was so important to me, I realized that there was value in surrounding myself with people who understood my struggle. The Kamloops chapter of the MS Society of Canada became an important contact for me. I got a call one day in 2006 from the coordinator there who wanted to set up an outreach meeting in Williams Lake. I could assist her with that and so we organized the meeting at the seniors' centre in town, one late September day later that same year. When I walked into the meeting room, I was stunned at the number of people there, even though I knew from my list of telephone calls to invitees that there are a lot of people with MS in Williams Lake. Wheelchairs, walkers, and canes filled the room and crowded around the long conference table, but the part that shook me the most was seeing an old high school acquaintance and a girl from a younger grade that I barely knew. I recognized Jack, who, like me, had been on the high school track team. I recognized Tracy, who, like me, had played soccer, although she was a much better player than I ever was. The unfairness of MS hit me hard that day. Why must young people, active, athletic and *nice* people, be struck down with MS?

Shaken as I was, I was also plain mad. "This disease is NOT going to get the better of me," I promised myself. It was a spontaneous and heartfelt determination. I was stunned when everyone looked at me and clapped. Apparently, I had spoken my thoughts out loud. I had made that promise to myself, out loud, surrounded by new friends, crowded into that seniors' centre meeting room.

I continued to stay in touch with the MS office in Kamloops and eventually started to write a column called "Rural Perspectives" for their monthly newsletter. It was a column about living with MS in a rural setting, and I wrote it from 2009 to 2011. The co-ordinator for the MS chapter in Kamloops informed me my column in the newsletter had a large following. I was triumphant: I was a writer! Adjusting to life post-diagnosis was no walk in the park, but I emerged from those first years not, as I had feared, with a lesser life but one more full. Those years were not without their losses, but I was surrounded by my loved ones and I had discovered a new confidence and success in myself as a writer. I thought I knew everything I needed to in order to keep making it through.

It's Getting Tougher

We must accept finite disappointment,
but never lose infinite hope.
—Martin Luther King, Jr.

Of our three children, Sam is the child who is closest to nature, and he is the one who often disappeared for walks in the woods on his own. His love of nature didn't extend to our ranch animals though, I was disappointed to note. It was Lexie, who—in true little girl fashion—developed a crush on horses and horseback riding in 1996 when she was about four years old. She would pull on a pair of little white cowboy boots that someone had given her and, with a baseball cap perched on her small head, would go over to the corrals and ride one of the large ranch horses around in circles, in the sunshine. Her chubby little legs were too short to reach the stirrups and I would watch with a grin, thinking back to my own childhood rides on our patient old ranch horses, Blanco and Rebel. By 2006, these kinds of memories were bittersweet; they seemed to be all I had left of riding.

The next few years seemed to be frequently full of bittersweet memories for me. Although warm, tender moments with my children and my husband abounded, I was slowly finding that life post-diagnosis was becoming more challenging. In 2008 I quit the *Canadian Cowboy Country Magazine* column after four busy years. The excuse I used was that I couldn't honestly write about living and working on a ranch when my mobility was slowly becoming so impaired that I couldn't even ride a horse anymore. In truth though, the loss of my riding ability and my slowly decreasing mobility was making it difficult to stay positive about my life. I remembered my long-ago dream of the airplane crash. I felt like "I AM" hit turbulence and fell from the sky. My confidence broke apart and I spent days on the couch in the living room feeling sorry for myself. My spirits were so low that I barely had the energy to channel surf the TV and I started avoiding answering telephone calls. I didn't want to talk to anyone. Even my writers' group and the support of close friends wasn't enough to shield me from the fear and attacks of insecurity that come with MS.

Since 2004 I had been running along our ranch roads to keep my legs strong and my strength up, and in the two most recent years, I had been part of the family relay team in the Dave Jacob's Memorial Relay Run in Williams Lake in June. My section of the run was one kilometre, and with

Ben, Sam and Tom, we formed a formidable family team. Now, however, in 2008, I had to drop out of the team. The fact that I couldn't run was upsetting in its own right, but I was also upset because I knew my participation was important for our team's chance for entering the family division. I didn't want to ruin my family's day. It wasn't that I was a good runner, I wasn't, but we simply needed four people on the team to cover the distance.

Thankfully, Lexie—or "Legg-sy" as we had taken to calling our now long-legged, athletic daughter—took my place with enthusiasm. I settled for the role of support driver, driving team members to their various relay drop-off points and picking them up at the other end. It was a crushing disappointment for me. Even when our team, the Redl Runners, won the family division and I was taking their team photo, I was sour about the lost opportunity. I know full well this sounds petty, and there's nothing pretty in self-pity, but I was in a dark place at the time. I missed the early morning fresh air on the run, the camaraderie and friendly competition from the other runners and the feeling of being fully alive as the blood pumps through your chest and your heart seems to beat in rhythm with your footsteps. Running, like dancing, was a way to positively connect to my body and I felt like I was left with only negativity and an aching loss.

Plain old envy reared its ugly head in my life in those days, too. I didn't appreciate being the one who had to sit on the sidelines and watch other people do things I used to do. This is difficult to admit, as it happened to me for many years, but if someone told me about a great hike they did in the mountains or the wonderful day they had skiing, it made me quite jealous. I used to love being active outside and an envious little girl inside me sat down and cried while she felt sorry for herself.

Of course, I also knew that feeling sorry for myself wouldn't help anything. Despite my almost overwhelming feelings of frustration and loss, I knew I still needed to be active and feel like a useful member of society. This had always been the case when I was healthy. Even before the MS diagnosis, it was important to me to feel like an active contributor. Driving to town once a week to write with the writers' group while the kids were in school and I had a few free hours in the day or selling beef at farmers' markets for our ranch wouldn't have been enough to guard against my steadily growing fear of being "just a housewife" once the children no longer seemed to need me. Solitude, being at home with nothing important to do, just made those fears worse. I was afraid I would grow old and feeble before my time. I was afraid I would be a burden.

Thankfully, even though my confidence was wavering on those days when I was alone at home, my fear was strong enough to lift me off the couch and away from *The Oprah Show* on TV and launch me into other, admittedly random, endeavours. One of these first endeavours was taking swimming lessons in the pool in town. I felt like I was getting fatter and flabby; my body didn't like being inactive. Since 2008, I had been working out at Curves, the local women's gym, but the workouts weren't going well. My MS symptoms get worse with heat; when I warmed up, I staggered, which made my workouts at Curves often more an exercise in frustration than anything else. I decided to try swimming instead because when I swam I didn't heat up. Plus, I reasoned, a fall when you're already in the water is just another splash, right? MS was not going to get the better of this body!

It had been a long time since my childhood days swimming with our neighbours in Rose Lake. I hadn't even really learned the front crawl, so I decided I needed a refresher. I booked a private half hour with a young lifeguard who was between Lexie and Sam in age, and I finally learned how to really, truly swim. It took a good month of practice, but I reached the stage of swimming lengths in the Williams Lake pool. Most times I swam for an hour.

I was happy with my progress; I thought I was still somewhat fat but not in the least flabby. Tom started coming with me a few times a week on the excuse that he wanted to stay fit. That's the excuse he used, but I know my husband well enough to disbelieve it. He doesn't like water. He was keeping an eye on me. I know he worried I would fall on the slippery tiles in the changeroom or on the pool deck.

Swimming wasn't the only thing that I did to keep myself busy. I also continued to help out at the farmers' markets. Tom was supporting his brother's dream of selling organic beef. In 2008, Tom and I started dutifully loading up a trailer with freezers and driving an eight-hundred-kilometre, three-day round trip every other weekend. We would eventually do this for at least ten years to access farmers' markets in southern BC. Tom was always the driver, putting thousands of kilometres on our faithful Dodge truck—the same truck that took us across Canada. I rode along in air-conditioned comfort because my left leg just wasn't strong enough to push the clutch around anymore. I enjoyed riding along, soaking in the beautiful scenery of these trips, but particularly the rugged, brown mountains and raging, foamy waters of Cayoosh Creek on the Duffy Road around Lillooet. I also loved reconnecting with the friends I'd made among the vendors and customers at the markets. Slowly, however, I had to admit it was taking a few days for me to recover from these busy weekends. I continued to go when I could, but when it was really hot in July and August, I stayed home. The heat made my MS feel so much worse, and I didn't have the energy to enjoy myself when it was too hot.

Not only was I fighting against the depression and negativity that come with MS, I was fighting against the physical realities of the disease. 2008 was the last year of not using a cane and the last year I was able to sometimes pretend to myself that I wasn't disabled, at least not yet. After all, I didn't need a cane to walk! Nature is an unforgiving mirror, though, and 2008 was definitely a year of many harsh reality checks as the losses continued to pile up. One day that winter, my friend Verena came out to the ranch to go for a walk with me. It had snowed the night before and we marched along for a couple of kilometres through fresh, deep snow before turning around to go back. There, in the snow on the road behind us were our tracks. Nature-as-mirror showed me that Verena's tracks were straight and sure, even and true. My right bootprint was steady and straight as well, but my left bootprint swung out in a neat half-circle with every step I took so my tracks looked like a crazy sewing machine stitch. My body was already compensating for weakness and foot-drop in my left leg.

Learning to recognize and then accept my limitations was difficult. I was determined to keep on with my gardening efforts in an attempt to stay active and keep my sanity. Gardening was, as ever, a joy and secret obsession of mine. Unfortunately, gardening is very physically demanding and especially challenging here in the cold and stony soil of the Cariboo. It was slowly getting to be too difficult for me. In 2009 I realized it would only be a matter of time before I had to give up my vegetable garden. Even my tiny flower garden was getting to be too much hard work. I started leaning towards planting less-flamboyant perennials rather than my bright and cheerful annuals. It was simply getting tougher for me to kneel down and stand back up while I was planting new seeds. It's the bright, colourful annuals that I love the best, however.

One of my favourite flowers is the sunflower. The sunflower's bright, cheery face always looks happy, especially on a grey, rainy day in mid-summer. Whenever depression threatens to strike and I start to feel sorry for myself, a big, bright yellow bloom can lift my spirits in no time.

One August day I sat on my knees weeding the flowerbed across our front lawn. I was scratching out weeds from between the sunflowers when I heard a rustling in the tall grass at the edge of the lawn behind me. Thinking it was just the cat, I ignored it until two rather roly-poly brown bear cubs came tumbling out onto the lawn. My first thought was, "Where is the mother bear?" In my panic, I didn't even stop to consider how I was going to get to the safety of the house until I had the front door knob already in my hand. I don't think I staggered across the lawn that day. My body, for all its challenges, is still often able to do exactly what it needs to.

Although there have been frightening and extremely painful moments during this journey, like falling on a cement floor and bashing up my knees and hands while trying to get up, there have also been encouraging times when I am reminded that I am still strong. Strong enough, when the chips are down. I never did see any sign of the mother bear. Perhaps she was taking a moment too, to enjoy the sunshine and not worry.

Although gardening was getting more and more difficult, I relearned other ways to commune with nature. I could just sit on an old stump in the woods and listen. It's something I started as a child and picked up again as the MS slowly advanced in the mid to late 2000s. As a girl, I had a special, private spot in the leafy green trees behind our ranch house and I used to sit there and just listen, watch, and observe nature with all my senses. In the seventies, I attended church services in the summer conducted by travelling missionaries, Shantymen, spreading the word of God to isolated communties. In my days of attending the Shantymen's Church, I got to thinking of this time in nature as talking to God. An atheist might think of it more as a meditation, but now I'm thinking it was just me, communing with nature, and in the late 2000s, I reactivated that practice.

I spent as much time outside as I could, even with the MS and not always just sitting on a stump. The children were with me a lot of the time and one of my best memories is of Sam running headlong through the thick, dark-green brush beside a ranch road, with bright orange flames leaping up behind him. That memory is not as terrifying as it might sound at first. Something I have loved to do since I was a little girl—and a love some of my children seem to have inherited—is setting fires. Fire was used in the old days by people like my father and grandfather, and still is used today, to clean up areas of grass and brush in the spring and fall when the ground is either still damp from old snow or just covered with a new snowfall so that the fire can't spread. On that particular day, Sam had climbed into the trees where I couldn't go anymore to a small brush fire his father had started. Sam set a thick, dry fir branch on fire and then ran over the snow-covered ground with it to another pile of brush that was ready for burning while I watched him run.

Ben and I still laugh about the early spring day when Tom came in from working on the ranch to find the two of us leaning on garden rakes by the garage door. We were surveying our day's handiwork and in between the spring-green trees all around us were acres of blackened grass and charred remnants of old, dead stumps, and a fine grey ash was still raining down on everything.

"What the…" Tom started, and Ben gleefully interrupted him, "One match, Dad. Just one match did all this."

I had learned that old pioneer way of "spring cleaning" from my own father, and while I wasn't fast enough to run for the water hose or bucket to put out a stray spark anymore, Ben was, and he was my insurance that my spring cleaning efforts wouldn't get out of hand.

Not all the children were that enthusiastic about fires, though. When Lexie was a teenager, she still muttered about the day I sent her running to get some water in her little yellow sandbox pail to douse a couple of sparks that had gotten dangerously close to the house. She was too small as a toddler to manoeuvre the heavy garden hose and I was already too weak. That was the last time I tried to set fire to anything, much to Tom's quiet relief and Lexie's more vocal utterances.

I still cherish the memories of "spring cleaning" on the ranch, though, and the sight of a ditch or meadow covered with dead grass makes me itch to toss a lit match into it. There is a feeling of awe I still always get when I think of nature's great, consuming power and how it is so easily brought to life in flame.

Although I'm a Canadian Cariboo woman through-and-through, German traditions run deep in my over-achiever psyche, and they are particularly strong around Christmas time. It occurs to me that while both gardening and meditating in the woods are ways of communing with nature, certain old European cultural traditions encourage that communication too. They are all ways to strengthen one's spirit through bonding with the earth. Many of the old German traditions I grew up with continued to play a role in my life as a mother, much as they did for my mother when I was little. A winter day in late November is always dedicated to making the annual Advent wreath. When I was little, Mom would make one every year when

Advent season rolled around and it was always exciting. The Advent wreath means Christmas is just around the corner, and for the next four Sundays, there will be candles and baking with mugs of delicious hot chocolate in the middle of the afternoon. As a child, it was always the four red candles that drew me and fired my imagination. Barb and I took turns blowing out the candles. It was a huge pleasure to watch, once I was a mother myself, my own children Ben, Sam and Lexie take their turns blowing out the candles. Although none of my children speak German, they learned the Advent verse that Barb and I took turns chanting in the warm house in front of the glow of the candles, while the beautiful, deadly white snow piled up outside:

> Advent, Advent, ein Lichtlein brennt
> Erst eins, dann zwei, dann drei, dann vier,
> Dann steht das Kristkind vor der Tuer
>
> [Advent, Advent, a little light glows
> First one, then two, then three, then four,
> Then the Christ child is at the door.]

Tradition, or the power of ritual, of history, is important to me. Tradition, too, relies on repetition, on certain things being the same. I remember how determined I was to be able to keep things the same those four or five years after the diagnosis, which became especially more difficult when I started using a cane in 2009. By then I found walking without assistance too precarious. I tromped through the cold, drifting snow under the winter black, sleeping conifers on the ranch behind our house while I muttered to myself and occasionally cried out loud at the difficulty of staying upright while harvesting branches from our fir trees, when I could find them, and the horribly sharp-needled, stiff spruce, when I couldn't. Once I was back inside the warm house, I twisted the branches into a glorious wreath topped with four red candles and a gold star. Tom loves the wreath and now that the kids are gone, I carry on the tradition for him. And for myself. As long as I can. At least, that's what I told myself.

Because of the weight of "tradition," and my own unforgiving expectations for myself, I felt I had to harvest the branches myself for many years. It's just recently, in 2014, that I got smart and decided to take things easy. As the old-timers used to say, "there is more than one way to skin a cat," and there's more than one way to make an Advent wreath. I actually bought a pre-made wreath in Williams Lake at the grocery store. They had a huge display of Christmas trees and a smaller one of fragrant fir wreaths. I could see it wasn't as thick and luxurious as the wreaths I used to make from branches I harvested myself, but the wreath looked OK once I had decorated it with the traditional gold stars and red ribbons and set it in the middle of our table.

Using a cane — or canes — whether I was inside or outside was an adjustment. I tried to stay positive about it. I still remember my 2011 visit to Abbotsford. Unlike me, my sister Barb left her ranching roots behind. I love seeing how happy she is with her husband Darren and her daughters Erin and Kayla in their tidy neighbourhood, but it does reinforce to me that I am not, despite my time in Germany or Victoria, a city girl. Barb's neighbourhood is full of cookie-cutter houses with grey roofs fronted by small squares of green lawn. Admittedly the lawn is green year-round, even when in December our fields have disappeared under a blanket of white, but I love the Cariboo with its four seasons and wide open spaces.

That December in 2011, I had stopped in to deliver Christmas gifts. It was a typical grey, West Coast day. The girls were entranced by my cane, which I introduced as "Theodora, who helps me walk." The girls seemed to accept my explanation. Kayla was six years old and Erin eight years old. Kayla was a whip-smart, outgoing kid who was always busy, busy, busy. Erin, a platinum blonde, blue-eyed, gorgeous little girl, was also smart but shyer than her sister. I was faintly sad but mostly quite touched to notice they were both very careful around me, especially when I was close to the stairs. The steep, carpeted stairs down to the entrance of the house from the living room were plain scary to someone like me who was starting to wobble. I tried not to worry about what would come in the future—how I'd handle stairs once I was in a wheelchair, what the girls' reactions might be then. One day at a time, I decided. I held the railing tightly with both hands, praying there were no loose splinters to come off and stick in my fingers while I side-stepped up and down the stairs.

Barb, not only her daughters, offered comfort. She continues to be an awesome sister and a great support. She keeps prodding me to fight and not give up in our occasional emails to each other or in Facebook messages.

Back in 2009, Ben was twenty-one, Sam nineteen, and Lexie seventeen, and I could hardly believe how independent they were. Time has a way of marching on, regardless of how we view it and how we endure our own struggles. Stubbornness drove me even more than fatigue in the first years of dealing with MS. I decided I wanted a paying job and to get myself out of the house and off the ranch when the children no longer needed me. As the disease slowly shackled my abilities to move around freely, coincidentally, it progressed in time with my children growing more independent and needing me less. In fact, one by one they were slowly growing into adulthood and leaving home. Ben had already left and was studying engineering at the University of Alberta. Sam was preparing himself to follow in his brother's footsteps and Lexie was eyeing up the bright light of graduation with great anticipation.

Finding work in the real world as a retired stay-at-home mom is difficult enough, but it is nearly impossible as a handicapped person. It takes a special employer to hire a disabled person and to have faith that the person will work out for the best. But it's been well-documented that any prejudice against disabled workers is unfounded. According to a recent article in the *Chronicle Herald*, and in a host of other studies and papers, handicapped people usually prove to be very good employees, whether that handicap is mental or physical.

After looking for a job for several months, I found a job at the Williams Lake and District Chamber of Commerce. Fortunately, the place was managed by a woman I'd known for years, whose daughter also struggles with MS. Claudia was not only quick to overlook my handicap, she was also quick to hire me. It didn't hurt that I knew her from years past and had even briefly taught her German in a night school course. Claudia knew me pre-MS and didn't judge the way I walked or my tired appearance. I have always appreciated her faith and confidence in me. I worked at the Chamber of Commerce Tourism Information Centre, and it was, for the most part, interesting work. It was strange to go back into the work force after being at home raising the kids. I sometimes found it quite frustrating to be working with nineteen-year-olds but, to be fair, we had the same skill set when it came to the job. Life experience doesn't count for much when you're applying for jobs outside of the house. Nevertheless, when the tourist season got busy and we had people lined up at the counter to speak to a visitor counsellor, the line-ups were formed in front of me. I wonder if folks naturally gravitate to people with life experience when they want to be sure they're getting competent answers. That's unfair to the nineteen-year-olds who could answer questions about our region as well as I could—then again, maybe they didn't know the region as well as I did. After all, Tom and I and the kids travelled every inch of the Cariboo and a lot of the Chilcotin.

Part of the job for the Chamber of Commerce was writing profiles of businesses for the chamber newsletter. This meant travelling through Williams Lake and interviewing business owners and operators. I got to know a lot of Williams Lake business people this way. I also got to know which businesses are handicap-accessible, which is something I was, sadly, starting to watch out for. A long, narrow flight of rickety stairs leading up to an open office over a sales floor made me pale-faced with fear. If that banister on the stairs, the one I had a death grip on, ever gave way...

Despite the dangers of unfamiliar staircases, it was good to get out of the house. Not only did it give me a reason get out of my ranch hand's jeans and t-shirts, it made me feel a sense of purpose. With my confidence in my physical strength wavering, I needed another outlet. With the kids more independent, I didn't want to feel relegated to the role of "retired housewife," especially as I was increasingly feeling inadequate in the skills I felt were required in that role. Although I was never a Martha Stewart, I did love her magazines. She embodied the housewife's dream, but I could not ice my cupcakes like she does... or carve my Hallowe'en pumpkins the way she does... or, whatever. For some reason, this had never bothered me much before. Now it did. MS was making me feel bitter about all sorts of aspects of my life. Fall fairs abound in this part of the country and they are the place and time when the Martha Stewart wannabes shine with their sewing, preserving, and flower-arranging abilities. I was competent in these areas but I never excelled. Never have. Although I knew my heart just wasn't into making perfectly piquant cucumber relish — although I knew my strengths lay elsewhere — I found myself focusing on what I couldn't do. I was finding it more difficult to stay positive.

Part of the MS fight is physical. I fought back by training at Curves, by swimming, by gardening, by walking. Part of the fight is mental. Part of that fight is emotional. I had to fight back that way too. I needed to remember the bright sunflowers, the beauty of nature, and the many other things that MS could not steal from me.

One day, a woman with MS in a wheelchair asked me, "Are you stubborn?"

"Incredibly," I answered truthfully.

"Then you'll be alright," she replied.

I'm not too stubborn to learn from other people though. It wasn't until an elderly friend in Williams Lake told me a tiny part of his World War II war story that I finally realized I need to change my entire attitude towards MS. He had fought for the English in the war and spent time in Germany afterwards, helping the German people recover. His sympathies for the German people amazed me and humbled me. I could not imagine feeling any sympathy for the people who shot at me. That would be like being grateful to this disease, MS, wouldn't it? It would be trying to be thankful for what the disease is teaching me. Somehow, the analogy clicked—I had a new way of looking at my life. I would regard this disease as something that picked a fight with me and is losing on the battleground where it counts. The battleground is my soul, and I would not surrender. I would not stay negative. I would keep fighting, keep loving myself, my family, my friends, my land, and my life.

THE CURE,
OR MAYBE NOT

*A ship is always safe at the shore—but that is
NOT what it is built for.*
— Albert Einstein

In November of 2009, Tom and I were helping out his
brother, as we so often did, by selling beef at a market in
Williams Lake. It was bitterly cold, so I was glad the annual Medieval Market was held indoors. Hosted by one of
our local high schools, this Christmas market was called
the Medieval Market and the theme was, well, medieval.
We vendors were dressed in cloaks, tunics, long dresses
and leggings. Inside the high school gymnasium, where
the market was held, the bright overhead lights showed
the myriad items on offer. Most vendors brought arts and
crafts, like jewellery, sharp knives, soap and blacksmithing
items like trivets, but some brought food: homemade jams,
honey, coffee and, of course, our beef. Despite the market
space being full and somewhat crowded, the market was

quiet. Maybe all those cloth items for sale—bright scarves, patchwork quilts and knitted sweaters hanging everywhere—muffled the noise. I was squirming; I'd been manning our vendor's booth for too long and my bladder was full, threatening to spill over. I tried to ignore my body's complaints while my friend stood in front of our vendor's booth with a delighted grin and told me she had just heard on the radio that the cure for MS had been found. Liisa, who I had known for years, was standing in front of us with a broad smile and bright eyes, almost laughing while she told us her news. I was afraid to get too excited. I was nervous to let myself think about the possibility of a cure too much, but all through that day people came trooping up to me in bursts, beaming with the good news. Suddenly, the hard-fought-for feeling of peace that I thought I had achieved was gone. That fragile feeling of serenity and acceptance had disappeared, popped like a rainbow-coloured soap bubble with the sharp stick of reality. I'd been through so much to achieve that feeling: denial, bargaining, anger, grieving. Learning to live with multiple sclerosis was an emotional roller coaster, and I thought it had plateaued, but now there was another steep climb.

The Medieval Market ended. Tom and I went home and I tried get my bearings again. Before I could make sense of this whole new opportunity, however, a fellow MS-er, someone I knew from Williams Lake, went to India for treatment for Chronic Cerebrospinal Venous Insufficiency (CCSVI treatment), which is also known as Liberation Therapy. Others were planning on going to Costa Rica or Poland, and my comfortable world of peace and acceptance was flipped upside down.

Within the month of November, I had started doing my own research. I read medical reports and countless blogs posted by other people with MS and bookmarked pages and newsfeeds to do with CCSVI on the internet. CCSVI, the apparent cause of MS, could be cured by performing angioplasty on veins that had somehow narrowed. This, in turn, would cure the disease. At least that was the claim.

I was desperate for guidance from the Canadian medical system. The system, however, even the MS Society of Canada, the one I had been fundraising for, was quiet about this new promise. In frustration, I lashed out with one of my columns for the MS newsletter, blasting them for the silence and lack of hope, of help.

Through my research I learned that Dr. Paulo Zamboni, a physician from Ferrara, Italy, claimed to have cured several people of MS by enlarging the veins that drain the brain so that blood can no longer pool in the brain and deposit metals like iron. Therefore, he concluded, there is no further injury to the brain of MS patients, the scleroses stop forming, and in some cases the damage already done is reversed. He further claimed that MS is not just an autoimmune disease; it is at least partially caused or exacerbated by twisted or blocked neck veins. Dr. Zamboni had performed vein-enlarging surgery on many MS patients, including his own wife.

Although the premise sounded a little hokey, considering all the things I'd been told over the years about MS, and I didn't want to be naive about a "miracle cure," the procedure seemed to actually work. Dr. Zamboni had cured every one of the patients he'd operated on, including his wife. Although Ferrara, Italy, where he lived and worked, is a long way away from an isolated cattle ranch in Miocene, BC, I found myself wanting to go see him. First things first though. I needed an MRI showing the veins in my neck. That was not as easy as it sounded. There was no MRI unit in Williams Lake at the time, and there was no way for me to access the one in Kamloops. Neither my doctor nor any neurologist in Kamloops would order an MRI just to check my neck for proof of Dr. Zamboni's premise. The public MRI units and even the private ones in Vancouver were booked for months ahead and there was not enough staff to meet the demand of MS patients clamouring for MRIs around BC.

By this point, in the winter of 2009, I was walking with a cane a lot of the time and I knew full well my mobility was only going to get worse. I was bitter about my whole situation once again. I had to accept that things were deteriorating for me around home and in my life, in general. A lack of patience was making itself known and I harangued the MS Society offices in Kamloops with my accusation that they had neglected to take action on their members' behalf. To give the staff full credit, they did respond to me and let me know that the national society was looking into the matter.

Even the UBC MS clinic heard from me when I called to find out what they were doing about "the cure." They told me they were spearheading a trial into Dr. Zamboni's technique. That was all I could have expected from them anyway, I thought, still mightily frustrated with the lack of action shown by the Canadian medical establishment.

I wasn't the only person with MS who was frustrated at this lack of action. Once a month, a group of people suffering from MS met in Williams Lake. It was an offshoot of that first meeting I had gone to at the seniors' centre the day I had inadvertently blurted out my intention to win this battle against MS. The "support group," as we called ourselves, met monthly. When news about Dr. Zamboni's discovery hit, the excitement in this group was palpable. So was the frustration when we all realized we would have to pursue this opportunity on our own. There would be no help from our doctors or our neurologists.

We were all desperate for news of the new procedure and desperate to find ways to have the procedure done. Even those people who had been in clinical trials of promising new drugs in years past, drugs which had not turned out to be the answer after all, were excited about this new promise. Those who did travel to other countries to have the procedure done paid heavily for the opportunity.

"We cashed in our life savings," said one caretaker, whose spouse was in a wheelchair. "How could we not take the chance?"

A couple of months later, in the spring of 2010, during a trip to Vancouver to see my neurologist, she said, "Wait a year, see what happens, this is a new field and I don't recommend it for anyone with MS."

In Williams Lake later that spring, my family doctor simply said, "Ew, angioplasty in a vein?! That's dangerous."

I knew, though, that despite the medical profession's concerns, Canadians with MS were flocking to private clinics abroad to have the angioplasty procedure done. I didn't want to be left behind and this situation brought out the gambler in me. My decision to undergo CCSVI treatment was a very, very personal one. On the one hand, I didn't like the thought of having someone push a balloon-on-a-needle through my jugular veins. On the other hand, I didn't like the thought of someone pushing me in a wheelchair in a few short years. I weighed the odds: one-third of people who have had the CCSVI procedure done have experienced immediate, great improvement in their MS symptoms, one-third experienced moderate improvement, and one-third experienced no improvement at all. I decided to take the chance, even if the Liberation Therapy no longer looked like the sure cure for everyone.

Tom wholeheartedly supported my desire to go for the procedure. One morning in spring 2010, when I was still doing research on CCSVI on the computer, he appeared at my side and said, "If you want to do it, let's do it!"

I think I was more hesitant than he was to commit that amount of money on a gamble. We talked about the prospect at length in the living room that morning. Sitting on the floor in front of our fireplace, I picked at a white leaf in the pattern of our carpet over and over, raising and smoothing the short, thick pile of carpet as if the movement of my fingers could lead me to the right answer. I kept wondering, what if? What if it could help? $20,000 is a lot of money to potentially waste on a fix that doesn't work. But what if? What if it works? If it worked, I would have energy again. I could ride again. I could ski. I could run. The list of "could's" was tantalizing.

Tom assured me he was willing to spend the money to take the chance. That morning I saw in him the same strength I had noticed in that dance hall twenty-five years ago when I was only twenty-two and he was twenty-nine and we had our entire marriage ahead of us. We had no idea, back then, what the obstacles would be. We certainly did not anticipate that twenty-five years from that first date, we would be heading off to Mexico to a private clinic so that I could receive a controversial new treatment for a disease whose cause is still unknown.

"You sure got the short straw when you married me,"

I said, feeling sorry for myself and for him that morning.

He didn't say "don't be silly" in words, but it was there in his tone when he said forcefully, "I don't see it that way."

I chose a clinic in Mexico because my research showed it to be a lovely, modern facility and because it was much easier to get there than to fly to Ferrara, Italy. We arrived in Mexico on November 22, 2010, over a year after I had first heard about "the cure" and we were immediately taken to Sanoviv Health Resort, just south of Tijuana on the Baja peninsula. We were going to stay for a week, the length of time specified by the "cure" program I had signed up for. I was trying to notice everything, taking mental notes of the flowers that bloomed so profusely even in November, the deep blue ocean beside us, and the white adobe buildings of the resort. This attention to detail was partly my own artist's temperament cropping up but it was also out of a sense of duty. Just before we'd left, I'd received a very nice letter in the mail from a lady who lived in Lillooet, BC, and who was a regular follower of my column in the MS newsletter. She, plus about another dozen people, had signed up for email updates about my progress in Mexico. All of them were MS patients themselves, and they were eager to follow my progress but they were still unsure whether the cost of the procedure was worth the risk they would be taking. I felt like a live specimen on a lab table but I also felt strangely gratified—if this is how I can help people now, I thought, then so be it. Verena, bless her heart, had given me a diary book to record my experiences in before we left, and I referred to my diary daily as I sent email updates back to Canada.

The entire experience was interesting—not pleasant, not unpleasant, just interesting. Tom claimed Mexico has a distinctive smell. I'm not sure as I couldn't decipher one in particular but I know the air felt different there. It was denser, warmer and more comforting on the skin than the thin, cold, dry air in the Cariboo. It was almost hot the day we arrived and I was grateful that we were there in November, not earlier in the year when the sun would be higher in the sky and the heat fiercer and more unbearable. As it was, I understood fully why so many Mexican ladies wear loose white blouses in that heat. Sanoviv is a beautiful, holistic resort set up on the Baja peninsula for medical tourists. Doctors, nurses, nutritionists, masseurs, even a dentist were all on-site. It was November, but tropical flowers were blooming around the resort in all shapes and sizes, their bright pink, orange and purple flowers providing brilliant splashes of colour against the green grass of the hotel's lawns. The resort had about four main buildings for housing and treating guests besides the hotel and dining room: library, doctors' offices, spa facilities, a gymnasium and more.

At Sanoviv, Tom and I were both treated like royalty. I guess that's what money does for you. The food was plain and simple, fresh and fabulous. It was dairy-free, gluten-free, and it was basically salads. There was little to no meat other than the occasional piece of fish and everyone who went there—as either a patient or a guest accompanying a patient—lost weight. In my diary I noted that I was going to miss decaf coffee and desserts, while Tom was going to miss potato chips and Doritos. During that week, while pitying the people who were walking around dealing with pounding caffeine withdrawal headaches, I was dealing with my own lesser headache. I quickly learned that decaf coffee still contains some caffeine.

Sanoviv prided itself on being allergen-free. The floors throughout the resort were a warm beige-coloured tile, easy to clean. Tile extended into the spa rooms where it was a peaceful blue colour and even out onto the pool deck. Three pools were available to patients and guests: a plain lap pool and two thalasso therapy pools with hand rails and lifts for handicap access. We were given plain "uniforms" of unbleached cotton to wear: pants and a loose tunic top and plain sandals. Our toiletries were provided by the resort. They consisted of natural soap and natural toothpaste. The soap was plain and unscented. The toothpaste looked and smelled like wet beach sand. It tasted OK though when you brushed your teeth with it. There was no makeup for ladies; everyone was fresh-faced.

In fact, one morning I whispered to a new friend at the breakfast table, "How did you manage to find eyeliner?"

She grinned ruefully, "They're tattoos. They were done when I was seventeen."

Not only our diets were adjusted at Sanoviv, but our sleep routines were also. We were in bed by 9:00 pm as nothing electronic would work in the resort after dark and, oddly enough, we slept deeply and well despite the early bedtime. At 5:30 am, quiet classical music was piped into our room to wake us up with the sunrise. It was an insistent but gentle alarm clock, goading us into starting our healthy day.

There were water stations set up throughout the main hotel building where we could refill our resort-supplied water bottles whenever we wanted and we were encouraged to drink a full two litres of water every day. Several times a day, young women carrying a large tray full of tiny paper cups of wheatgrass juice would come by and insist we take a cup. Tom gamely took his cup and drained it, claiming it wasn't that bad. I looked at the rich green, thick liquid sloshing gently in my cup and told him forthrightly, "It smells like lawnmower clippings." A nearby potted aloe vera plant was the discreet recipient of my wheatgrass juice and from then on I avoided the tray-bearing young ladies. Whenever I glimpsed one coming, I would head in the other direction as quickly as my ungainly, floppy, healthy sandals would allow.

Every guest wore the same uniform and had a name tag with a coloured dot beside their name. We quickly learned that people with green dots on their name tags were there for the CCSVI treatment and those with red were there for cancer treatment, and we also quickly made new friends. Everyone was in the same boat: physically ill or accompanying a loved one, suffering from sugar and/or caffeine withdrawal, and marvelling at how fast we started to feel well.

My admittance photo, taken on the first day, shows a lady who is a bit overweight: my face slightly flushed, as if I'm retaining fluid, and a fresh crop of pimples along my jaw line. Those were the result of stress, I was told. I believed it because I hadn't had a breakout since I was in my teens and the thought of the procedure I was about to undergo was weighing heavily on me. I wasn't stressed though. No, I was flat-out terrified.

The Liberation Therapy procedure itself was done on November 25. Tom and I jokingly referred to the procedure as "roto-rootering" because of what was done. It was performed in a hospital in Tijuana, which sounds like the punchline to a joke, but in this case it wasn't.

I remember being awake for the entire procedure and listening to the doctors say, "Breeze Haydee, breeze. Stop breezing." English wasn't their first language. I breezed and I held my breeze (breath) and wished for the best. Oddly enough, once I was on the operating table, I wasn't scared anymore.

Feeling the balloon probe go through my heart wasn't a walk in the park. Neither was the intense pressure when the probe reached a narrow spot in my vein, just below my collarbone, and I felt the balloon inflate, trying to widen the vein. I thought my head would pop off from the pressure. It was supremely uncomfortable, like having bricks piled up on my neck, one at a time until I almost passed out from the weight.

The lead surgeon liked the Beatles. I remember that — while I was lying on the operating table listening to McCartney sing, "Hey Jude," — I was thanking my lucky stars he wasn't crooning about "the long and winding road" as the probe snaked through my veins. I also really like the Beatles, so that may have helped me to be more relaxed as well.

The procedure widened one place in the vein just under my collarbone and opened a valve in the other vein, a valve which had grown too long and was stuck in the closed position. When it was over, I was wheeled to a quiet, green-curtained, post-op recovery room. The bright-eyed, always-smiling doctor from Sanoviv came in to see me.

"Well?"

"I don't feel anything, other than an electrical-type tingling running up my legs."

"They're waking up." Then he told me that the narrowing in my vein was most likely congenital: I had been born with it.

"Will it close up again?" I asked. "Will the other vein

be blocked by that extra-long valve again?"

He shrugged, smiled, and patted my leg. There were no promises.

After that there was just an ambulance ride back to Sanoviv. I'm sure the flashing lights and siren were used solely to impress the pretty, young nurse who attended me in the back of the ambulance. The ambulance driver was a young, good-looking man, obviously single.

Once back at the resort, I was required to spend twenty-four hours flat on my back with a sandbag lying over the incision site in my femoral artery. Somehow I managed to sleep that night, lying in a dark room at Sanoviv with only the sound of the ocean rolling in outside the black windows. I had never used a bedpan before but I wasn't allowed to get up, let alone move. My incredibly loyal, loving husband emptied the bedpan for me. That night I learned the true meaning of love. You have to love someone to voluntarily empty their bedpan, don't you?

Tom was with me every step of that journey. We attended mandatory meditation classes together and he didn't scoff at them once, although I know he doesn't believe in that sort of thing. We attended mandatory gym classes together and even mandatory cooking classes where we learned how to make healthy salad dressings and salsa. Together we walked the walking path, a half-kilometre loop through green-grey, salt-sprayed native grasses beside the ocean. In fact, the only time Tom left my side was to get a massage that he sorely needed. I couldn't have had a more attentive or trustworthy companion.

The morning after my surgery, after the sandbag was taken away, I was in the shower and I noticed that not only were my feet warm, I could feel the hot water from the shower on and around my feet as it made its way to the drain. I hadn't been able to feel any surfaces I had stepped on for several years now as the nerves in my feet had stopped transmitting signals to my brain. Tom had been the first to notice this as he started to lose tickle fights. My feet just weren't ticklish anymore. I debated against sharing this news with him, solely for that reason.

Later that day, we joined some other guests in the outdoor thalasso pool to the amazement of some of the resort staff. They were wearing parkas and shivered with cold whenever they stepped outside.

"Are you from Alaska?" they would ask. "We had guests from Alaska who swam in the winter." I proudly shared my Canadian roots.

I walked back onto the airplane bound for home seven days after arriving at Sanoviv, my collapsible cane folded up in my shoulder bag. I still limped slightly but I had a lot more energy than I had had in years. My diary entry for that day read: *loved it here but glad to go home. It's time to go to work.* I couldn't believe my luck. The procedure had worked for me.

DISAPPOINTMENT

Courage doesn't always roar. Sometimes courage is the little
voice at the end of the day that says,
"I will try again tomorrow."
—Mary Anne Radmacher

Before I went to Mexico in 2010, I had been using a cane to walk around on level surfaces in buildings and on sidewalks, and I had been using poles to walk outside. I took long walks on the ranch as long as I could; I also eventually started to write about those walks, sensing that they would not continue for too many more years once I needed poles for balance and support on the ranch roads

Life after the procedure in Mexico was different. I was delighted to leave my cane and even my poles behind when I went for walks out on the ranch, in the fields behind our house. In November, after coming back from Mexico, the fields were covered with snow. I stuck to the roads that had been ploughed for feeding the cattle. Over the years, I had always kept an eye on the ravens that populated the ranch and congregated around the cattle-feeding areas in winter, looking for a free speck of grain. I had also long amused myself by calling out to the ravens, matching them croak for croak when they sounded annoyed or imitating the long, oddly musical trill they sometimes made. This one day in November I remember particularly well because a young raven appeared in the blue sky above me and croaked. Surely, I thought, it didn't recognize me. Nevertheless, I croaked back. Flapping those black wings a little faster, it flew lower and ahead of me, and then it turned back and flew right at me. The raven was close enough for me to see its bright eyes when it tucked a wing under its breast and did a barrel-roll onto its back in mid-air. While I stood with open mouth in utter wonder, it nonchalantly righted itself and soared over my head and off into the distant thick, dark evergreens behind me with a final croak. I felt like I had been welcomed home and back into my rightful life.

We had long since stopped doing the huge family Christmas dinner as Tom's parents had passed away and other, more distant in-laws were dying off—but immediate family still brought stressors with it for me at Christmas-time. This year, however, the year after the CCSVI procedure, was the first year in a long time that I felt I had the energy to handle it all. I moved around the house, the ranch, even Williams Lake, like I had two hundred pounds of cement lifted off my back. I had my old life again and it felt great.

Christmas was an easy time that year. As usual, it was soaked in traditional German festivities and Canadian turkey. Lexie was still at home, in grade 12, but Ben and Sam were away at university, and it was a treat to have them home for the holidays. We all enjoyed visiting together, finding and then decorating the tree, playing games with the extended family and, of course, eating. I love shortbread and Lexie helped me bake it that year. Luckily Sam and Ben like to eat it too, or I would have eaten it all myself. I seem to have no willpower around Christmas shortbread.

Christmas passed; 2010 turned into 2011. I continued my work at the Chamber of Commerce. I also continued to write for the MS Chapter of Kamloops's newsletter as a featured columnist. I wrote about the Liberation Therapy and MS for other Canadian magazines, too. I joined online support groups for post-CCSVI patients and tracked my progress on their website graphs. I answered blog questions and even agreed to be part of UBC's tracking poll, answering questions about every three to six months on how my progress was coming along. I wanted as many people as possible to have CCSVI treatment for MS, fully believing it had helped me.

The Williams Lake and District Chamber of Commerce has long had a policy against hiring staff, or electing directors to chamber positions, who are involved in politics. The way I grew up and my continuing love for the environment around me naturally drew me to the Green Party in politics. When I was asked if I would run in the 2011 election as a Green Party candidate, I agreed without hesitation. It meant leaving my Chamber of Commerce job and travelling the length and breadth of our 225,310 square-kilometre Cariboo-Prince George riding while I campaigned, but I had my old energy and stamina back and that was no problem for me. The federal riding of Cariboo-Prince George extends from near Williams Lake in the south to Prince George in the north and Vanderhoof in the west. Cities and towns in this area include Williams Lake, Quesnel, Wells, Prince George and Vanderhoof. Voters in the Vanderhoof and Prince George area tend to vote Conservative while voters in the Cariboo tend to lean towards the NDP and I knew this would not be an easy election for a Green candidate, who historically comes in fifth in this riding on election day.

One of my most memorable moments of that whole campaign occurred during a debate in Wildwood, just north of Williams Lake. We seven candidates were seated at a long table in the school gymnasium for the debate and I noticed a tall woman in a long, red coat near the back of the small crowd seated in front of us. After the debate, she came up to congratulate me on how well I did and how long I had been able to stand up, without support, during an Indigenous prayer. It was the "friendly gynaecologist" from years ago—the same woman who had started me on my journey towards a confirmed MS diagnosis. I was oddly pleased to have her see me in what

I felt was my natural role as a strong woman, rather than a disabled one.

I did well in that election, in that historically strongly Conservative riding, coming in a solid and respectable third place on election day. This was helped in large part by appearances by Adriane Carr and Elizabeth May of the Green Party, who seemed delighted to come and campaign with me for a couple of days. I was glad I'd had the energy to meet that challenge head-on, but the whole experience was still exhausting. All that work, stress and effort took a lot out of me. I decided to hang up my campaign signs and not campaign again as I was exhausted for weeks after the election and had, during the last weeks of the campaign, gone back to using my cane. I wanted to go back to being just me: mother, wife, and rancher.

In 2011, by the time of the election, my children were all grown. Ben and Sam, of course, were still busy at university and although Lexie was still at home, she was busy with grade 12. I decided to once again find a meaningful job in town, following my foray into politics. Although running for the Green Party had not given me the winning result, I had come out of the experience feeling more secure in my convictions and with a greater sense of self-respect. I needed to do something active and positive.

Slowly, oh so slowly, I was learning to treat myself and my body with respect. I do not have the stamina or strength to do physical work and I am too strong-minded to take direction from other people, particularly when I don't agree with them. A job where I could contribute to society, without feeling like I was somehow inferior to anyone else, was what I was looking for.

I had a new confidence in being a working woman off the ranch. Earlier, in the spring of that year, I had seen a sign up on the door at my gym, Curves: *PT help wanted.* I thought, "Why not?" I was looking for a job and I hadn't had any luck anywhere else I'd applied in Williams Lake. I'd been very open about having MS and, in return, had been told bluntly that I couldn't handle the job. One of the ironies of my working life was that when I started work fresh out of university with the Canada Employment Centre, my job was to find work for disadvantaged people under the Career Access program. Visible minorities, disabled people, women, and youth were considered disadvantaged when it came to the job market. Now that I was disabled myself and would be eligible for that program, it no longer existed. I was lucky to have the opportunity to apply at Curves. Sue, the owner, knew me well and knew about my ongoing struggle with MS. Her sister had MS too and had just had the CCSVI, or Liberation, procedure. Sue hired me. My job was to clean the circuit and coach women on the machines and I even did the occasional workout myself. The pay was minimum wage but I didn't care. I found that I was, surprisingly, really enjoying my job and the social contact. In fact, the regular social contact became invaluable to me. I missed being needed as much as I was when the children were young. Some of the work at Curves became almost a replacement parenting job for me. The children may not need me anymore, I reasoned, but customers like Bernie do.

Bernie is my age physically, but about six years old mentally. She is just slightly shorter than me, at about 5'6" and she is quite a bit heavier. Her hair and eyebrows are dark and her skin would be white, if she didn't spend so much time outside in the wind and sun. Bernie is unapologetically herself. She talks a lot and loudly, and she's very straightforward in her communication. In other words, you always know what Bernie is thinking. To me, that's the best thing about Bernie. She is totally honest. There is nothing duplicitous or dishonest about her. She'll tell you if she likes something and be equally forthright if she doesn't. Politeness is not a strong suit of hers, but you can always depend on her to tell you the truth. She can read and she has a decent memory and she's not shy to tell me she loves me. I started giving her a ride home after work but then she started coming to Curves early and hanging out there just to be with me. Sue had sold the business to my new boss, Anne, who was also lovely to work for but who quite rightly set out limits for Bernie's presence at the gym. Eventually, Bernie's membership got rescinded. It was a relief for me because she would impose herself on me while I was trying to work and she would get jealous when I was helping other customers. Still, I always gave her a ride home because she continued to wait by my car on days when I was at work.

In my first months on the job—while Sue was still my boss—a typical afternoon shift at work would go something like this:

The door-bell chimes. Bernie comes in and stomps by me wearing a carefully constructed scowl.

"Hello, Bernie."

She turns, her lower lip quivering. "Those people aren't very nice to me."

"Who, Bernie?"

"The café owners. They don't want me to help them anymore at their café. Well, fine, I won't help them." Her face clears and now she wears a big smile.

Holding her arms out wide, she says, "Heidi, I love you this much." It doesn't stop there though. She comes around the reception desk for a hug, her problems with the café obviously forgotten.

"You going to work out with me?" she asks.

"No, not right now, Bernie. I have work to do here. I have files to update. You go ahead without me."

"Oh." Her face falls into gloom again.

"Don't forget to wash your hands before you go on the circuit." I escape back to the desk and the files that are stacked up, waiting for me. Ten minutes later I glance up and scan the circuit. Bernie is working out, bouncing on a cardio pad with a peaceful expression on her face.

By this time, it's time for me to start cleaning the floor. I can't help but smile. Bernie's attitude, even her presence, cause a lot of people to feel uneasy, but she came to fill an important role in my life. I feel like a caretaker when I'm with Bernie.

Of the few jobs I have had outside the home over the years, the job at Curves was the best, and I think that was solely because my boss was a woman. Both Sue and Anne understood the pull of family commitments and were grateful, in turn, that the staff were flexible enough to fill in for each other. At that stage in my life, I would not have done well working for someone who is inflexible or pulls the "big boss" act.

For about half a year I was working on the high caused by that Liberation Procedure and I walked, worked, and coached. While Sue still owned Curves, I had a shift every day and I was working full-time as a member of our productive Canadian society. When Anne bought the business, my job went part-time and I was grateful. The long hours at work were a bit too much for me. Under Anne's watch, I took an online course to be a certified Curves weight-loss consultant and a hands-on first aid course at the university in Williams Lake. The first aid course was day-long and very tiring but still, it felt good to have my normal life back. I was working and living as a regular member of society without the stigma of being handicapped. Little by little though, the disease crept back into that life and I took a few falls. Some of them happened at work when my foot drop would cause my running shoe to snag a loose spot in the carpet or a stray cardio pad on the circuit. Eventually it became obvious to me what others had seen coming for so long and I grabbed a cane for support. Again.

"Thank God," one of the members said the first time she saw my cane. "You need something. You scared me every time I saw you walk without anything."

Anne was solidly reassuring, saying she didn't mind if I made my way around the gym with a cane.

"Heidi, you're an inspiration to the other members," she told me repeatedly. The members, indeed, seemed to not notice my cane at all. I really don't think it surprised anyone. At first, it didn't bother me too terribly much, even though I'd hoped the Liberation treatment would have given me a bit more time with a reversal of the disease. Truthfully, a mischievous imp in my soul took delight in hanging a paradoxical cane on the wall beside the fitness circuit when I did my own workout. The fact that I could do my own workouts still, unimpeded, buoyed me up.

My love for my children buoyed me up too. Lexie graduated in June 2011. She is a beautiful young woman (yes, that's a proud mother speaking). Her grad dress was a rusty brown colour, which sounds horrible, but it looked spectacular against her pale skin and dark red, long hair. Tall, slim and naturally friendly, she had no trouble finding a date for her graduation prom and as a proud mother, I put on a leg brace to guard against accidental foot-drop-caused falls and went to the prom as an assistant. I, together with Ben and Tom's help, staffed some of the fun activities set up at the "dry grad" prom put on by our local school board in an effort to keep new graduates from drinking and driving. When I watched Lexie, so confident and poised, for a fleeting moment I remembered what it had been like for me when I graduated from high school; back then, I was healthy and had no problems, or even thoughts, of MS. Did I miss that time? Would I go back? No. For all the difficulties that I've faced, I wouldn't trade my life for anything—being the mother of such an intelligent young woman and her two equally wonderful brothers reminds me of how privileged I am.

I continued, too, to find great solace in nature, and I was still walking as much as I could on our ranch. Whether it was in winter or summer, nature provided me with an energy boost and helped to ward off dark and gloomy thoughts. My natural bent for writing came into play and I kept a diary, noting excerpts like this one from February 26, 2012:

> I walked down to the Gopher Rock in the Barley
> Field today. I would have liked to go further, but

it snowed heavily two days ago and the road isn't ploughed so even with yak-traks on my boots I was slipping a bit and stumbling in the ruts made by Tom's truck tires. Harry-the-poodle enjoyed the walk though and had no trouble, skipping along, jumping and following his nose. Tom caught up with us when we were on the way back to the house, on his way back from working in the woodlot. It's a beautiful day today, clear sky and sunny.

Later, in March, I wrote again.

There's a stiff breeze from the south-east today and I didn't stay out very long. I also didn't have to wear longjohns because it's 5 C. The sun shining off the snow and ice on the road made it very hard to see in the glare, but I did see a wondrous cloud above me. It was a thundercloud, all dark and grey on the bottom where it was perfectly flat. On top it was puffy and lumpy, like pieces of light gray and white cloud all gathered together and dropped haphazardly onto the flat surface below. Sunlight highlighted the top of the lumps in yellow. There was a slit in the cloud about halfway along the bottom and rain was pouring out of that slit.

One of the walks that resonated with me most powerfully happened on a deep autumn day on the ranch. At the time, I didn't write about it because it resounded so strongly with me that it became part of my soul and I knew I could never forget it. I can imagine it perfectly now: I walked into the woods behind the hayfields and the experience became magical. I liked to walk all the way to an old house on a neighbouring piece of property and it was a good five- to six-kilometre round trip. On this particular day there was a slight breeze blowing golden and yellow leaves off the poplar trees. As kids, Barb and I would chase around the trees by our house with buckets trying to catch as much "money" as possible, but we never had any luck with our bare hands. On this walk, on this day, a large yellow cottonwood leaf floated down in front of my face and pretty much landed in my outstretched hands. Two grey whiskey jacks perched, one on each side of the gate into the wood, and stayed there as I passed. They made me think of sentinels, watching me pass through into a land of magic—a warm land sweetly scented by the autumn woods and as full of magic as the imaginary world of icy ferns and trees that the frost painted on my childhood window. The woods smelled like new wine and the sky above me was a bowl of bright blue, protecting my world.

Multiple sclerosis is a sneaky disease, though, and a strong opponent to battle. While I had thought in earlier years that constant fatigue was the worst symptom, in later years I have come to realize it is depression that is the heaviest burden to bear with MS. Depression can creep up on you and blindside you, seemingly out of the blue, and walking in the woods was not enough to shore up my soul's defences against depression.

Fighting back against the feeling of being useless, I started thinking I should be paid for the work I already do, outside of my regular job. Unfortunately, neither the environmental newsletter I wrote for nor the MS Society could pay me for my writing work. With mixed feelings, I quit both of those volunteer jobs. I regretted giving up the MS Society newsletter column because there were people who enjoyed reading it, but I wasn't sure it was good for me to wallow in self-pity and write every month about my struggles with life.

Other than having multiple sclerosis and suffering from depression, my body seemed to age normally. While this should have been encouraging, I'd be lying if I said that aging thrilled me at all. I now need glasses for reading and for driving. I chose progressives to cover the wide range of my needs and I wear them all the time. While I don't mind wearing glasses too much—after all they make it easier for me to see—I find I mind the annual eye checkup very much. Part of that is the optometrist's insistence on putting eye drops in my eyes to dilate my pupils so she can check the entire back of my eye for macular degeneration.

She did it once and I felt so physically sick, so uncomfortably nauseous, that I've sworn off the procedure forever. Now, every time I go in for my annual eye check, I have a discussion with her where she argues that the procedure doesn't make one sick and I argue that it does. So far, I've managed to stay firm and my eyes are checked for macular degeneration through ordinary pupils.

I find that people in the health profession, whether it's chiropractors, optometrists or whatever, are quite excited to have a person with a serious, non-contagious disease come in to their practice. Whatever my problem is, be it a twisted muscle or floaters in my vision, it is viewed through the filter of multiple sclerosis and seen as a learning opportunity for student staff. I've contorted myself through various positions for trainee physiotherapists, chiropractors and masseuses, and my young optometrist could barely contain her excitement when she introduced me to a visiting optometrist who specialized in particular eye problems. The funny thing is, my eyes don't have multiple sclerosis problems. They're just ageing. Normally. The visiting optometrist reluctantly agreed with my amateur assessment after running a battery of unnecessary tests. It does seem odd to me to be making other people so excited about this disease. I wish I could be as thrilled.

Tom and I were very busy in 2012. Between my job in town at Curves and Tom's work on the ranch, we didn't take a holiday. In April 2013, however, we cruised to Hawaii on Holland America's *Zaandam*. I was using my cane a lot by then and that very fact was depressing. Actually, I was feeling pretty depressed by my lot in life and by the fact that I was still declining physically, so the cruise was a great distraction.

On the way down to the Port of Vancouver, a seven-hour drive, I noticed that the scenery was no longer as beautiful as it had once been. Not even the horses grazing in the fields we drove by were beautiful to me anymore. Hills, trees, rocks, horses and cows, even the mighty Thompson and Fraser rivers were all coloured in shades of grey. Depression was sucking the colour out of my world. The Hawaii trip that lay ahead of us that April, with its vibrant, tropical colours of blues, reds, yellows and greens, couldn't have come at a better time to remind me that there is more than grey to my life.

The *Zaandam* sailed out of Vancouver on April 18 for a seventeen-day cruise to, and around, the Hawaiian Islands and then back to Vancouver. The Vancouver home base for this cruise made it convenient for me and other Canadians to board this ship and partake in all the on-board activities. The convenience factor extended to people with disabilities, who were able to enjoy a wonderful, relaxing cruise with their families. There were wheelchairs, scooters, toddlers and grandparents galore. My cane and I fit right in.

The *Zaandam* is not a large cruise ship, by cruise ship

standards, but it absorbed and dispersed its cargo of people and assistive devices with grace. The first thing I noticed was the friendliness and helpfulness of the crew. Not once was I able to manoeuvre a tray of food through the buffet line; as soon as a crew member spotted me trying to handle my tray with one hand and my cane with the other, he or she was there with a friendly smile and gentle insistence, taking my tray and walking it to a nearby table. Partway through the cruise, I mentioned this courtesy to one of the staff and he informed me that they are all specially trained to help people with mobility issues.

I had no idea until this trip how large the Pacific Ocean actually is. I had looked at atlases, of course, and studied globes, but the enormity of that ocean doesn't sink in until you spend six days with nothing on the horizon except waves. The odd piece of garbage floating by was a lousy reminder of our planet's growing pollution problem but when I was sitting with my feet up in the ship's forward lounge, sipping a piña colada and looking at a world full of water and clouds all around me, the odd orange bucket or sheet of black plastic was a bright and easily visible reminder that nothing is ever perfect.

My multiple sclerosis still made me extra sensitive to heat. While I was initially leery of touring the Hawaiian Islands in spring's hot weather, my concerns proved to be ameliorated by life on board the *Zaandam*. Oahu, Maui, the Big Island and Kauai provided us with breathtaking scenery, and, although the heat did make me wilt, particularly one day on Maui, the *Zaandam*'s air-conditioned hallways, library, theatres and restaurants were always available to us while we were in port. When the days got warm in the Pacific as we headed south, the retractable roof would open over the pool and I spent hours in the warm water and reclining on the lounge chairs on the deck around the pool—always within easy walking distance of the food bar, of course.

In Honolulu we first found the wonderful hop-on hop-off trolley system that is now in place in major cities around the world. You jump on the trolley and ride it until you see something you want to look at more closely so you get off and a while later you get on the next trolley and continue your ride. We were sitting on the top deck of the trolley in the open air with the scent of tropical flowers mingling with traffic fumes when we drove by the Honolulu police department. The driver snapped a CD into the speaker system and suddenly the *Hawaii Five-0* theme song blasted around us.

Instantly, I was ten years old again, sitting in front of our TV in the old ranch house in Miocene, swaying and singing, "Bah, ba, ba, BA, BA, BA, ba, ba, bu, ba, bum." Yes, I'm older now and I'm handicapped, but that moment brought a strong young girl back to mind: a strong, young girl who loved life and loved *Hawaii Five-0*, the TV show.

Later, Tom and I strolled through a market where vendors were selling trinkets and souvenirs to tourists. It was a hot day under a cloudless blue sky and the market, with its paved walkways snaking between crowded tents hung with brightly coloured goods like shawls, beach towels, and jewellery, provided a little bit of welcome shade. It was noisy, bright and somewhat overwhelming. I'm easy to catch up to as I'm slow with my cane. A young man took advantage of this and thrust a small, gilded box at me. "This will cure you," he said.

If it weren't so ridiculous, it would be funny. Some people will prey on the handicapped or disadvantaged, trying to make a buck any way possible. This memory stays with me because I am not innocent of gullible belief in trying new things. I drew the line with this young man's trinket, but I have been buying self-help/self-healing books and experimenting with diets.

Besides reading self-help books in the library, I spent a lot of time in the ship's art gallery on that trip, admiring the paintings and studying the artists' brushstrokes and the colours they used. I think the art gallery, more so than even the inspirational books in the library, helped to lift up my spirits so that when we left the ship in Vancouver again, the city seemed to be a much more colourful and busy place than it had been when we had arrived over two weeks earlier. The trip home, too, showed me the colours of late spring coming to the land as the Thompson and Fraser rivers were blue in the sunshine and the sage-brush-dotted hills were a gentle green from spring rains. Closer to home the greens deepened and darkened as the boreal forest showed itself in the thick, tall evergreens of the Cariboo and Chilcotin plateaus.

My interest in self-help/psychology books stayed with me after the cruise, though, and I searched through the Williams Lake library shelves for volumes that might help me. Later that summer, for example, I worked on "Walking without a cane" with the guidance of a self-help book I wasn't sure I completely believed in. The process involved much mental work, much learning about emotions and realizing that I sometimes used MS as a crutch. The theory was this: I was using it to protect myself from doing things I don't want to do or am afraid to tackle or from situations I am afraid to be in and for gaining sympathy. I decided I must stop doing that. I needed to stop doing things like, for example, taking Lexie's boyfriend down to the shop to look at Tom's car and walking very stiffly with two poles. What was that? The boyfriend at the time wasn't all that interested in Tom's Mustang, but I used it as an excuse to show him that I needed protection because I can't walk well on my own. Was I worried about losing Lexie? If he was a threat that way, then I had just played the sympathy card. Terrible. Lexie is a grown woman with a right to her own life, I reasoned, and so am I. I'll never lose Lexie's affection and I can enlarge my heart to encompass a love of hers—a new boyfriend—so really, I didn't need him to help me in any way. I felt foolish. Then again, maybe all this New Age healing shit about emotions is just that—shit.

For the most part, I refuse to give up and let MS get the better of me, but sometimes I waver in my faith. One day, feeling low, I moaned to my friend Ann: "I'm going to be the old woman sitting in the wheelchair watching life go by."

Ann just laughed. "You're going to be the old woman sitting in the wheelchair bitching about something," she asserted.

I had to laugh too. I am not a passive person. I'm not content to watch life go by. I have to live it.

Shortly after that conversation with Ann, an article in *Macleans* irritated the heck out of me. The article bashed the "Liberation Therapy." I wrote the magazine a scolding letter, but it really got me thinking. The article concluded that CCSVI treatment didn't work and wasn't worth the expense that people with MS poured out to be "cured." It forced me to really consider how the treatment had worked for me. I knew on some level that I was doing better than I would have been had my MS followed the "normal" route and timeline. I had undergone this treatment in Mexico two-and-a-half years ago and since my treatment I was able to go back to work. In fact, I worked as a fitness trainer at a women's gym. I had to admit to myself that it is true that the treatment is not the cure for MS but I reminded myself that I knew that going in. Yes, as before, I still use a cane, but the procedure gave me a vast improvement in the quality of my life. I was trying to convince myself that the money Tom and I spent was worth it. Looking back now and taking off my own rose-coloured glasses, I see that the Liberation Procedure gave me about a year-and-a-half's worth of actual reprieve from the disease's inroads. I had the surgery in November 2010; by 2012 I was using my cane again, and by later that year, I was slowly starting to feel the same way I had before the surgery was completed—depressed and fighting to stay positive. The physical decline caused by progressive MS continued, but I still somehow felt better off than before the treatment. For the most part, I was able to keep the depression at bay. It was still a battle, but I seemed to be winning it more easily than I had prior to my CCSVI treatment. That was probably simply because I had more energy and I was willing to take on challenges in my life once again, specifically, working at a job.

I often have a little talk with myself when I do face challenges. Each talk always starts with, "Face the facts, Heidi…" One day in the summer of 2013, it went, "Face the facts, Heidi, you're not enjoying being in the community band." Ergo, I wrapped up my flute and sent it to our niece Erin. Little Erin got my flute as her Christmas gift. She's twelve years old now and according to her band teacher, via her mother, she's a strong flute player. Gifted, even. Good. May the flute be good to her. She looks like a little angel playing it with her big blue eyes and long, white-blonde hair. My fingers were slowing down and my heart was never in it anyway. The last few weeks of being in the community band, I felt like I played the flute only out of fear of letting things go, letting abilities go because if I let them go, I may never get them back.

So, I didn't play the flute anymore. My world just pinched in a little tighter.

I fought against that feeling of pinching, though. One way I coped with a world that seemed to be shrinking physically was to try new endeavours that I could accomplish. I started to sing in Angela's Just for Fun Choir. My friend Angela hosted a party at her house when she turned fifty. I met some of her other friends there, friends from all the different things she is involved in. Two of them were talking about singing and how they don't know how to sing. Angela started a choir for women who plain love to sing. The choir sounded good. I joined it. Now, I sing happily on- or off-key (I'm not sure which it is and I don't care) with the choir on Fridays. We're called Just for Fun and our subtitle is A Joyful Noise, which is what we produce at times. Even though I do say so myself, I sing well. I love to sing. It turns out I have a naturally high soprano voice, though it is a bit weak in volume. My singing helped push against the pinching caused by giving up the flute.

Singing is pushing out the boundaries of my shrinking world ever so slightly.

That Christmas, in 2012, we sang Christmas carols for the season and Angela had the German speakers (there are four of us) organized to sing one of the verses of "Silent Night, Holy Night" in German. It's a small group of voices that do it but I have to admit we sounded good. Although that was over four years ago now, I still go and sing with Just For Fun when I can and I still enjoy it as much as ever.

It stuns me at times when I'm faced with the fact that I have had influences on people throughout my life so far. I am particularly touched to think of a couple of neighbour girls, Kristina and Erica. I had taught them and their little twin sisters Laura and Emma during the years when I first became active with the writing group. Their mother had hoped I could help them to connect to their heritage more by teaching them German. I remember trying to make the lessons fun, and I was touched that, so many years later, we had a positive relationship. In 2013 Kristina shocked me by telling me she wanted to paint our house for us and the proceeds we paid her were then going to be donated to MS research.

"Your house will be my MS project," she said when she took on the Student Works house painting contract as a summer job. She and her sister Erica also drove down to Kamloops with me that same year and together with a few more of their friends, we formed a team and walked in the MS Walk. It felt a little strange to see all those young people wearing a "Walking for Heidi" sign on their backs. More than a little strange. It was humbling and... weird.

Kristina has grown into a beautiful, mature woman. She and her crew came out and painted our house right before we put it up for sale. They did an awesome job. Kristina followed through and put all her proceeds from that job towards MS research. Wow. Wow that she would even think of doing that. I'm glad she's a close friend of Lexie's, because she has a big heart and a good head on her shoulders.

Angela, too, has stayed very close since I developed MS. She supports me in any way she can. In fact, she and I first started travelling down to Kamloops together to participate in the big MS Walk, which is a major fundraiser for the MS Society and she was also part of the "Walking for Heidi" team. It's always pleasant to walk alongside the Thompson River in May. May is summer down in Kamloops while it's still the dirty, tag end of winter here with ragged pieces of snow banks sullenly melting among the drifts of winter-dead grass. Down by the Thompson River though, the early leaves are out in May and the sweet scents of garden flowers drift over the crowd of pedestrians and wheelchairs on this walk.

Angela and I had been going to this walk for a few years before Kristina and her friends joined us. I could never figure out why I suddenly couldn't walk well whenever

Angela and I gathered with the other MS walkers at the start line. I couldn't walk without stumbling, limping or dragging until we left the walk and headed for the mall to do some shopping before driving home. Three years in a row this happened to me. I didn't realize I was the only one who noticed this until Angela said to me one year that being at the walk felt like diving into a cloud of gloom that clung to every person there. Despite the beauty of the Thompson River, the uncertainty surrounding the many anxious participants was palpable. Angela felt the miasma of pathos and despair keenly and while it didn't affect her physically, it was clearly affecting me.

"You're Heidi Redl?" The question was posed by a woman who overheard me registering for the MS Walk one year. It turned out she was a regular reader of my column in the MS newsletter. She loved the column, she told me. That was sure a bright start to the MS Walk that year.

The children's friends, the children themselves, and their young lives and adventures keep reminding me that my life is not over yet, not by a long shot. Tom and I watched from a distance as our three children flourished and then graduated from university. Sam's university graduation in April 2013 was very much an epiphany—another turning point for me. I wasn't walking well at all, in fact my foot dropped, causing a fall. I took a train from Kamloops to Edmonton, where Sam was graduating. In the dining car on the train on the way there, I took a headlong nose-dive. Some strangers helped pick me off the floor and dust me off. I felt them watch me closely as I staggered, on shaking legs, to the nearest seat. It wasn't fun at all. But watching Sam graduate with First Class Honours near the top of his engineering class, now—*that* was fun. He was one proud lad and so he should have been. Tall, dark-haired and thin like his dad, blue-eyed and handsome, he's quite the guy. Tom had driven my little blue Honda Civic up to Grande Prairie where Sam was working to pick him up and sell him the car. Together they drove down to Edmonton and met up with me. After the ceremony, Sam took us back to the train station and he drove himself back to work at Grande Prairie, and Tom and I had a leisurely and enjoyable ride back to Kamloops on the train. With Tom travelling with me on the return trip, I didn't have another fall, but it was very much on my mind and I was very careful with every move I made. In fact, I was so careful that I whined, "I'm starting to move like an old lady." I knew I could seriously hurt myself if I didn't take more care.

Once back on the ranch in Miocene, I put off getting a walker. Finally, though, I conceded that I needed one. It felt like a kick in the teeth. The walker is such a symbol of disability and, unlike with Theodora, my trusty cane, there's no way to hide it behind my back.

I used the walker for about six months in public in

2013, but later that fall I got my wheelchair. It was a relief, in comparison to the walker, because I'd become so unsteady it was nice to be able to just sit down and by then I was used to being "the disabled one." The process of degeneration took place steadily, insidiously and mercilessly, over the timespan of about four years from the time I first started to use the cane.

Mentally, I held on though and kept fighting. Although I was slowing down physically, I stayed active in my mind. The kids still needed their mom's advice from time to time and I loved being asked for help. Specifically, I could help Lexie out with her university work as she earned her English and anthropology degrees. Sporadically, she would ask me to look over a poem she had written for English or to help with some archaeology research that needed to be done online. It gave me a sense of being useful, because of all the things that I still have going for me, I value my intelligence the most. I also value being able to communicate with people.

Every day I am so grateful for the internet. It connects me to my children and even to the rest of the world. Suddenly I didn't feel so isolated, living at the back of the ranch. The internet, Facebook, and email are life-giving social connections for people, especially disabled people who can't navigate the physical world.

My job at Curves, however, still required my ability to navigate the regular highway, let alone life's metaphorical highway. Living at the back of the ranch, forty-five minutes from Williams Lake, I relied heavily on my little car to get me out and about. It became my physical lifeline to the rest of the world and, as such, I loved my little car. It was a bright blue Honda Civic that sipped gas, rather than sucking it. It was also low to the ground, however, and by 2013 getting in and out of it started to be a problem. I needed the car for my sanity though, to get me off the ranch and into town, where I could work at a real job; a job where I could still contribute to the world.

My legs grew weaker with each passing month, despite the procedure in Mexico and despite my stubbornness. Finally, I was climbing out of the car by holding onto the top of the door, feeling like there was a sack of cement tied to each of my legs. Tom insisted it was time to get a new car for me, one that I could get in and out of easily. A so-called "level-entry" car. We looked around at various options, but it was after a holiday in Victoria with my friend Ann that I realized the benefits of an SUV. Ann had got me to drive her around Victoria in her SUV, visiting the bustling Chinatown with its tall, narrow buildings and stunning red gates, having tea at the Empress Hotel while obsequious waiters offered us special Empress-blend tea, sitting beside the uneasy ocean at Cadboro Bay and driving around the city's sparklingly scenic ocean drive. Once home I was all fired up to find my own Honda CRV. Tom and I quickly decided those cars are ferociously expensive for us, but KIA makes a small SUV called the Sportage and it features level-entry. In other words, I could sit on the seat and swing my legs in to drive. Plus, it's automatic and, honestly, the clutch and my left leg weren't getting along well in my little Honda Civic. The Ford dealership in Prince George had a 2009 KIA Sportage for a very reasonable price and Tom and I drove up there to get it. Unfortunately, they didn't want the Civic. Fortunately, Sam did. The kid drove a hard bargain, though, and got the car for a real deal. I loved my new KIA, but I missed the mileage the Honda got. It made me happy, though, as Tom and I took the train back home after Sam's graduation that spring, to picture my handsome son driving off to work in the little blue car.

Even with my KIA, it took an increasing amount of effort to remain mobile. This effort encouraged me, once again, to reconsider my priorities.

So, in the winter of 2013, I started to paint. Painting was something I could do from my wheelchair. I've loved painting and drawing since I was a child and I seem to have a minor talent for oil painting. I'm pleased to report that my paintings sell well when I display them at farmers' markets. Spreading colours on blank canvases is sheer fun for me!

My artistic streak is growing and stretching these days to compensate for my physical body. As my strength fades and my muscles degenerate, it is interesting to see how the people in my life react to the new Heidi. The Heidi that walks with a walker or relies on a wheelchair and is starting to stoop like an old woman as her core muscles lose strength. My family has never wavered in their support. Sons, daughter, husband, parents, sister and nieces are there for me, helping however they can. They are a blessing and I love that I can rely on them. My friends are in the same category as they help me out however much I let them. That is to say, however much that independent streak of mine will bend. Acquaintances are a different story. Most people acknowledge my struggle and will hurry ahead of my walker or wheelchair to hold a door open or will scramble to pick up my dropped cane before I can bend down to get it. Others, well, I've come to the conclusion that they are so busy fighting their own demons that they can't acknowledge that I'm deep in a fight of my own and can't reach out to them. I've learned to laugh at things. For example, one night Tom and I went out to dinner with a couple who insisted on driving us in their truck. Tom's truck was still accessible to me because of the running board and the handholds that I could use to pull myself up into the seat. The truck that pulled up in front of me and my walker that day, however, had nothing. Just a thigh-high empty space between the ground and the seat.

"Jump in," I was cheerfully invited.

"I can't." I answered firmly, surprised at the assumption.

149

"You could if you wanted to," I was told.

What can a person do but laugh at that attitude? However, it still hurts. It's like saying to me that I am inconveniencing people with this disease because I want to. I want special attention and I don't really need the extra help I'm demanding with my cane or my walker or my wheelchair.

By the end of 2013, my world really was shrinking. Some of that shrinking, however, was very welcome — Tom and I decided it was high time to move into a smaller house. We bought an empty lot and began building a new, much smaller house just south of 150 Mile House. Our old ranch house was starting to seem pretty big with our kids gone.

After fifteen years, though, it was a lot of work to clear out the old family home. It took Tom a few weeks to finish burning boxes of old papers we hauled out of the basement in late February: income tax returns from the eighties, logging load slips from the nineties, all sorts of letters about the water case on the creek, documents and stuff nobody needs or wants or cares about anymore. If anyone ever wanted to research our lives here on the ranch for any obscure reason, I'm sure the government archives have copies of all the important things. They're probably stashed somewhere in Victoria. For me, moving meant not only packing, but cleaning. I cleaned the house thoroughly, every week as it slowly emptied out.

The days when I had enough energy to clean the whole house were unfortunately becoming few and far between so I treasured them—while I had once resented the chore, I now relished it. Fatigue was really knocking the stuffing out of me as there were days when I felt too tired to go do anything. I was sometimes too tired to even leave the house. That's where other people began to play bigger roles in my life.

Angela and I entertain ourselves every year for our birthdays, usually by going for tea at the Thyme for Tea Tea House. We are exactly the same age, born only nine days and about fifty miles apart in Germany. She looks great and when I complimented her this year, she, being the good friend she is, complimented me right back. She also made me promise never to give up trying to look good. I can see her clearly, trying on hats in the Tea House. Angela has a thing for hats and she can wear them well as the shape of her face and her short, white hair suit being topped by a chic, sporty little number. I don't like hats, myself, but I swear, as long as I can, I will try to stay thin, wear nice-looking clothes and make-up and look good. Even if that means forcing myself to leave the house. Even if it means forcing myself into the pool or the gym in an effort to at least stay fit, if strong is no longer possible.

Of course, as the MS advances, being strong physically has become a losing battle but I am reminded by centuries of philosophers that have gone before that strength can also be emotional. I like to think that I am still strong emotionally, despite sporadic crippling attacks of depression. I'm still here and I'm still fighting.

ACCEPTANCE

"If we believe that tomorrow will be better,
we can bear a hardship today."
—Thich Nhat Hanh

Physically, the easing of burdens enabled by the move into our new home in 2013 was much needed by the time that we'd sold the house we raised our children in and moved down just south of 150 Mile House. Spiritually, I was still working on accepting the fact that not only did others still need me but I needed others; however, I was starting to understand how much accepting my need for help came with its own host of anxieties. I depended on Tom a lot. By this time, I had reached my fifties and Tom was pushing sixty. Both of us, not just me, were getting too tired of the ranching life. We were also looking ahead at life as a person living with MS and a caretaker for that person. That gave us a different perspective on things than even those couples simply facing the fact of aging have to deal with. Dealing with my MS really is a two-person job. In any couple in which one spouse struggles with a chronic illness there is an inordinate amount of pressure on the caretaker, not only to take care of the ailing partner but also to take care of himself or herself. That's because, of course, if the caretaker falls ill or becomes incapacitated, both people are in trouble. I slowly came to realize my husband will not say anything when he is in pain. He doesn't want to worry me.

Unfortunately, Tom is not invincible. Over the years, Tom has had knee surgery to remove a cartilage that was damaged in early years of playing soccer. His knee is "bone-on-bone" now and I know he's sore. In 2012 he had shoulder surgery after finally relenting to getting the procedure done. Tom waited until he couldn't lift his arm over his head anymore before giving in to the need for that surgery. Even then, when I picked him up at the hospital afterwards, his sole concern was for me to make it to my routine appointment at the neurologist's office later that day. I was reminded, once again, how lucky I am to have married Tom. It takes a special person, I think, to put aside their own agenda and take care of their partner. If I had it in my power to reverse this disease of multiple sclerosis, I would do it for Tom now so he wouldn't have to worry about taking care of me as we both slowly age. I no longer feel the need to do it for myself as I'm in a comfortable place these days. I'm safe, I'm pain-free and I'm OK. I'm particularly OK since we left our isolated home on the ranch late in 2013.

ACCEPTANCE

I felt the change almost instantly. I loved that I was not faced with climbing stairs and the doors were wide enough to accommodate my wheelchair. I loved that our new home was far enough away from Miocene that snow, not uncommon even in April back at the ranch, came two weeks later in the fall and left two weeks earlier in the spring. The decision to move was a lot harder for Tom than it was for me. Moving, for Tom, meant giving up working with his brother and being part of a lifelong partnership. Because of the partnership, leaving the ranch posed a few issues for us, of course, involving family matters, but in my mind the benefits have far outweighed the irritants. *Que sera, sera.* I'm slowly learning to trust that life will turn out as it should. All in all, moving away from the family ranch and moving into our new house was liberating. It enabled me to start a new phase in my life. I had a suspicion that the stress of life on the ranch was connected to multiple sclerosis flaring up in my life. This could be totally wrong but I have learned over the years to trust my intuitions and suspicions. There is a strong connection for me between stress and MS symptoms. This is why, for example, I have a heck of a time walking properly whenever I go to the hospital or I know people are watching me walk.

I am grateful, however, that our new home is still unmistakably Cariboo. I am tied to this land and I don't want to leave it, even if I can't ranch on it anymore. Tom and I first made an offer on the new property south of 150 Mile

House when I saw it advertised in the newspaper. We went down and looked at the property, of course, but its location was what sold it to us in our minds. The view is absolutely spectacular. It's an ocean of grass and small, gentle hills like waves. In the distance towering monster hills surround the city of Williams Lake, which is hidden from our view behind a tall, brown bluff. The sky is an ever-changing painting and our view of it is unimpeded. We have a row of large windows along the west side of the house and the room that is enclosed by those windows is where we spend our days; often simply admiring the view. There is a small draw just beyond the fence that encloses our two hectares. The draw is home to several tall old poplars and aspens and, occasionally, a moose. I suspect that is where the deer who come to visit our new house often hang out.

The two-hectare lot is much smaller than what Tom originally wanted, but it is close enough to Mom and Dad at Rose Lake for me, and close enough to the ranch and the woodlot for Tom, who continues to work the woodlot. Plus, it's only a fifteen-minute drive to town. This benefit was one I particularly noticed right away. I love our new house's proximity to the highway. People can drop in at any time, and they do. They are going by and stop in for a visit or a cup of tea. It's quite wonderful after years of being isolated at the back of the ranch and not seeing a single soul outside of the immediate family to be so in touch with people again. I think I got my fill of being a hermit. Ann laughs at my description of myself these days as a "recovering hermit" and claims she is using the phrase herself.

Building the new house and getting it finished was extremely satisfying. With every sweep of my brush, I was spreading wood stain, whether it be on a log or on a window moulding. The outside of the house logs have two coats of Nano Light Honey stain, followed by a clear coat. I stained the south and east side of the house and Tom stained the north and west side. Inside, the logs have one clear coat and another half coat on the rounded top of the logs. The window and door mouldings are walnut brown Tuscan oil and the door and window frames are stained the Nano Light Honey. Our house is beautiful and I helped build it! That fact gives me such a sense of satisfaction. I love to contribute, to create and build things. That hasn't changed. MS hasn't touched my soul or my way of looking at the world. Depression, of course, is a different matter.

Of course Tom did the bulk of the work on the house. He spent over a month alone laying down our tile floor. Together we stained the door and window frames and finally, the well-driller came to drill a well for us. Unfortunately, in his first attempt he drilled a sixty-metre-deep dry hole but we got a good well, eventually. The water here is soft and flat-tasting. Ranch water, both when I was growing up and on the ranch where I raised the kids, was hard enough to walk on but it tasted good. This water is easier on the house pipes and probably our body pipes but I add lemon juice to make it taste like… something.

Life really was much improved in our new home, but it did come—as I said—with new worries, too. Even though I didn't have to worry about stairs, or fitting my wheelchair through doorframes, I did have to worry about Tom. Although he coped well with his sore knee and his sore shoulder, I was painfully aware that if Tom got seriously injured or ill for any length of time that I would be in trouble, too. This point was really driven home after Thanksgiving in 2013. Tom and I had gone down to Squamish and then Vancouver on yet another farmers' market and beef delivery trip. We stayed at an uncle's place in Burnaby on Saturday night and other family members were there too, on their own delivery/market lay-over. It was decreed we must have Thanksgiving dinner and one of the women set about cooking a turkey and the trimmings. I sat in my wheelchair and watched, unable to help in any way at all, simmering in my depression while I listened to the bright chatter of the family around me. I have never, ever, felt so useless. This from the woman who once single-handedly cooked Christmas dinner for twenty-three people!

When we finally got back home, Tom and I both hatched a cold from germs we had picked up at one of the markets along the way. I was able to rest. Tom, however, continued to push and to work, either on the ranch or in the woodlot, until his cold morphed into pneumonia. The pneumonia hit hard and laid him low. He was bedridden and so was I when that blasted cold of mine turned into the flu. There we were, sleeping all day, barely able to eat or sit up long enough to watch a short show on TV. At first I coped with my occasional need to move around the house, specifically to go to the bathroom, by pulling my wheelchair right beside my bed so that I could slide my legs out of bed and land on the wheelchair seat with my bum. Then came the fatal morning that my legs would not move. At all. I had to reach down with my hands, grab my knee and pull and then push one leg out of the bed and then the other leg to be able to fall into my wheelchair.

This is the next stage of multiple sclerosis: being bedridden and unable to move. It had happened to me. I lay on my back in bed and stared an ugly, and no doubt short, future in the face. And as I did that, I remembered the silver rod I used to imagine as a little girl. I imagined a silver rod ran through me and connected the sky over my head with the earth beneath my feet. I could grab onto that rod and lift myself up, whenever I had fallen down.

That miserable late-October day, grey sky bringing so little light to the bedroom where I lay unable to get up, I reached up and grabbed that silver rod and then I pulled myself up, pulled both of my legs around with my hands and pushed them over the edge of the bed, fell into the wheelchair and pushed myself around the house as hard as I could.

I wasn't giving up, not yet.

The year went on and Tom and I attempted to settle into our new lives at the new house as empty-nesters and watched our kids settle themselves into their adult lives. Ben finally screwed up his courage and applied for the job of his dreams with CN Rail. He's dreamt of working for a railway since he was seven years old and now he's a civil engineer; he's centred in Kamloops, just four hours away. As a mother, it felt, and still feels, so good to see him smiling and happy and confident in his life. He must be over six feet tall now as he looks down on me with amusement, but he's still thin, angular even. More and more, Ben reminds me of my tall, thin Opa, the one who was called "Turm" or "Tower" in his youth. Sam, too, has settled into life as an electrical engineer in Grande Prairie and seems to be happy. He's just shorter than Ben and is built slightly broader. He is one busy guy, working and keeping his hobbies alive. Sam still enjoys cooking and baking, gardening, and now he's added woodworking to his repertoire. Of all the kids, Sam is the one who looks most like me, although he doesn't like to hear that. Lexie looks a lot like my mom did in her early twenties.

Lexie graduated in 2014 with a double-major in English and anthropology. While she is trying to get her hair back to her natural colour, she's having a hard time figuring out what that colour is. It seems to have changed to a reddish hue on its own, under the brown dye she covered her original blonde with. She is having the time of her life travelling in Europe and has managed to keep her figure slim by staying very active in sports.

Luckily, Tom has an ability to think and plan ahead, that matches his generous nature. When I was first diagnosed, he decided we had to travel as much as we could while we were still mobile—that is to say, while I could still move. During our first summer at our new home in 2014, we went to the Mediterranean. It was a fabulous cruise. I never, ever really thought I would see Athens and Rome in real life, although I had dreamed about them as a child. Athens spoke to my soul, particularly up at the Parthenon where I thought I recognized statues from the stories I once read. Elegant and gracious, smoothly muscled and incredibly beautiful, they brought my childhood fantasies to life. Andromeda and Cassiopeia in the, well, stone! Rome was not as impressive. It was dirty and very crowded the day we were there as there were two canonizations scheduled for the following day. In both cities, the stone statues watched me impassively as I struggled along with my walker. Old European cities are not built for people who can't move on foot or bicycle. In the city centres, narrow cobblestone streets wind along between the buildings and the small, sharp cobblestones are a formidable barrier to wheelchairs or walker casters. There are also stairs everywhere! The people, though, make up for it. I had more people offer to assist me and hold doors open for me than I expected. It was like being at home in Williams Lake where people are also inordinately friendly and helpful when they see someone struggling along.

The day we were in Rome I was tired and it was hot. So I sat on my walker bench and Tom pushed me along. On our way back to our bus there was a steep hill and I was going to get off the walker and try to walk, to give Tom a break. However, before we really knew what was happening, five or six fellow bus passengers congregated around us and helped Tom push me up the hill to the bus. They didn't even pause at the curb. They all simply lifted me and the walker up onto the sidewalk. If I weren't handicapped, if I could move like a normal person, I would miss these things. That is to say, I wouldn't realize that people are essentially good and helpful. It makes me think back to when I was strong and able, and it makes me wonder if I helped others who were struggling along. I have to admit, I don't think I took much notice of disabled people or even people who needed help.

In 2014, I had long since given up sports, but I finally had to relinquish even walking with a walker outside as my sense of balance had really deteriorated and there is no easy way for me to get my wheelchair outside to garden. Gardening, however, was something I really wanted to hang onto. This proved to be a challenge. Deer resistant, drought tolerant, Zone 4 wildflowers that may grow here at the new house are limited to yarrow and coreopsis, which looks like a tall dandelion. In other words, weeds. That's not exactly a Garden of Eden collection of lovely perennials. I also wanted some plants that smell wonderful, like luscious roses or heavenly lilacs and while they are not weeds in any way, they could be naturalized to look spontaneous. Unfortunately, we're on a sunny, west-facing slope and the deer are an ever-present threat. I solved the problem with Tom's help. I filled two large half-barrel oak planters with soil and Tom set them up on our east-facing deck for me with a hose for watering close at hand. I filled those planters with tomatoes and surrounded the tomatoes with bright, sunny orange and yellow nasturtiums. The combination of warm sun, plentiful water and insect-laden air for pollination resulted in a bumper crop of tomatoes and a thick wall of nasturtiums spilling over the edge of each planter. It was a beautiful sight to my artist's eye. Mom added to the riot of colour on our deck when she brought down a planter filled with purple and white petunias, which I placed under my hummingbird feeder. And finally, I had enough tomatoes to make a tomato cake like Omi and Mom used to make.

Much to my delight, I also realized that I could of course paint flowers—and painted flowers are not threatened by deer in the same way that my garden would be if it weren't safe on the deck. I was able to indulge my fascination with colour and shape with a different artistic outlet. While I still have the use of my hands, I can create art. I particularly enjoy delicate watercolours although I am starting to dabble in acrylics and oils at Tom's request. I took a landscape oil painting course at the college in town. It was a one-day, all-inclusive course, and I painted a terrific mountain/lake landscape with a waterfall. Sam absolutely loved it so I gave it to him that following Christmas. One of my favourite little paintings of a group of pansies sold right away in Lillooet. Mike and Norm, who got married in August 2014 and who have the bakery tent beside us at the farmers' market, bought that painting and five others as gifts for their wedding attendants. It almost makes up for the smell of forbidden and fresh cinnamon buns wafting from their tent across the clear air to tease me in our little booth.

Despite my joy in the new house, our trip to the Mediterranean, and my love of painting, I was finding my deteriorating mobility hard to accept. The walker, and then the wheelchair, really did a number on my self-confidence. In the winter of 2014, after four wonderful years, I finally quit my job at Curves. Perhaps the hardest thing about quitting was knowing full well I may never work again. Now it's 2017 and I still miss the clients, my boss, and yes, even the trifling pittance of my paycheque. No matter how small it was, it was mine and I earned it. It always made me feel good to deposit it in the bank. Yes, I withdrew most of it as cash right away and yes, I then drove to the gas station and filled the KIA's tank and thereby spent all that cash, but hey—at least my job didn't cost us any money and I got some people-contact out of it!

I quit in October because by then the job was causing me a great deal of stress, although I couldn't pinpoint exactly why it was suddenly causing me stress. I think part of it was I was worried about another Cariboo winter coming and about the issue of getting the wheelchair through the snow to the door, then getting through the door and having to somehow wipe the wheels clean before going in to work. Although it came with sadness, quitting also came with a huge amount of relief. My boss Anne, though, has visited me a couple of times and a couple of times she's brought her sketchbook—it turns out she's an artist too and I enjoy her visits. She is more than a boss, she is another friend.

I didn't quit Bernie, though. Bernie still needs me to be her friend and so the two of us meet for coffee once a week for an hour. Then we go grocery shopping together. Bernie helps me with the grocery cart and I give her something to look forward to because, like me, she needs social contact. Like me, it's good for her to help and be helped. One of the things that MS has taught me is not just to be needed by others—but to accept the fact that I need others, too.

By this time in 2014 I was in a wheelchair and outings were getting to be fewer and further between, but I made sure, and still do, not to miss my weekly date with Bernie. It's not as easy to move around, but Tom built a wheelchair lift for my car and I can still drive. The effort was getting almost too great, but Bernie made me try, gave me a reason to try, and for that I was, and still am, grateful. She relies on me for her social time and I, in turn, rely on her for one weekly source of inspiration.

I tell Bernie she is my lucky charm. She's since glommed onto that and repeats it back to me at times. I swear it's true though. We meet for coffee once a week in a small coffee shop and Bernie is hard to miss: she's loud, enthusiastic and often inappropriate. People who sit at tables beside ours are often killing themselves laughing at our conversations.

My fifty-second birthday happened to be on our coffee day and so, as usual, I met Bernie for coffee. It also happened to be a snowy, grey afternoon and the coffee house was packed and full of noise and life. Bernie, being Bernie, let everyone within earshot know that it was my birthday. She bought me coffee. We sat and visited and looked at the newspapers and magazines she brought me, commiserated over my standing in the local hockey pool, et cetera, and all of a sudden a young man wearing a bright yellow turban came up to our table and said, "Did I hear it's your birthday?"

"Yes, it is."

"Happy birthday!" He dropped a gift card on the table.

I thanked him and he left. When I picked up the gift card it was for $20 to the Bean Counter, our coffee shop.

"Coffee is on me for the next little while," I told my Lucky Charm. Ten minutes later another, different, older fellow dressed like Tom usually is, in work shirt and faded, worn jeans, was standing beside our table.

"Buy yourself something nice for Christmas," he said, pushing a $50 bill into my hand. He left before I could even gather my wits together.

I was not only stunned by these events but shaken. "Bernie, I have to leave. This is freaking me out."

Lexie's response to this story when I picked her up from her waitressing job was understandable: "Mom, can I borrow your wheelchair?"

Lexie was being funny but she did give me some cause for reflection. I was now visibly disabled and an obvious target for kindness in my wheelchair. I strongly disliked being pitied, but at the same time, I thought, I was still being useful. I was now in the position of allowing people to give in to their best intentions. In this role, I would just have to put up with all the unasked-for kindness I was being showered with. People are generally kind and decent, I decided and hey—who is more obviously in need of a "lift" but the woman in the wheelchair having coffee with the mentally handicapped friend?

I do need to be lifted up, sometimes. Depression usually settles in with the change to winter weather, and things that I can't do bother me more than usual, like the fact, for example, that I can no longer go into the woods to cut branches for my Advent wreath. I know I've found good substitutes and I know that I have a happy, healthy family to celebrate and that is what's most important but it is difficult, sometimes, to stay positive. It's why I've taken to deliberately seeking out positive examples.

Paula Moulton and her partner Gary Lyness amazed the judges of the *Britain's Got Talent* reality TV show when they auditioned in 2012. As the wheelchair dancing duo, Strictly Wheels, they are the UK's first and only Latin Wheelchair Dancesport couple and the routine they performed for *BGT* earned them a live performance spot in the semi-finals. If I'm going to be stuck in this wheelchair, I decided, I at least want to dance in it. I love dancing. In fact, I would like to dance at my children's weddings. I have hope I will be able to do that. I have always loved to dance. I haven't forgotten that that's what first attracted me to Tom. He can dance. Dancing was one thing I was sure I would have to give up with the MS and the wheelchair— but I can still stand up and dance with Tom, sort of, as long as it's very slow and I have a death-grip on his shoulder and arm so I don't fall and drag him down with me. Paula Moulton's wheelchair looks to be the same model wheelchair I have, which is very lightweight and manoeuvrable.

One day I might need to convince Tom to give it a try with me. It looks like the guy only needs to watch his feet. You would hate to have some wheelchair casters roll over your toes!

By the winter of 2014, I had felt myself starting to get depressed again. There seemed to be no chance of dancing and I started wondering what exactly I'm here for, besides sitting in a wheelchair and breathing. In order to keep my mind busy and off my troubles, I looked for things to keep it occupied. I began to make lists. Lists of things I accomplished, like one month when I tried to accomplish three things a day:

- I picked up the tax disability form from the doctor's office and mailed it at the post office.
- I couriered my passport application from the post office.
- I dropped off Mom's woollen products for her at the Red Cross office.

- I joined Weight Watchers Online.
- I made guacamole for lunch.
- I did the dishes.

- I set up a recycling centre for the house.
- I had coffee with Bernie.
- I made lunch out of left-overs.

- I made breakfast.
- I made potato salad for lunch.
- I emailed Lexie.

- I laundered and changed the bed sheets.
- I made breakfast.
- I finished the deer painting.

- I vacuumed the house.
- I went grocery shopping with Tom.
- I went to an Elder College curriculum meeting.

- I made smoothies for breakfast.
- I introduced Verena to Angela.
- I attended the Miocene Christmas Market.

- I ordered canvas from Opus.
- I emailed Sam.
- I researched LifeLine.

- I visited with Mary and her kids.
- I watched Dr. Wahls's YouTube presentation.
- I lost one pound.

- I started a stew for dinner in the crockpot.
- I bought brushes and palette knives.
- I visited with Bernie.

The woman who once single-handedly hauled over two hundred books out of the Community Club library, swam fifty lengths at the pool, bought and washed three flats of berries, and started a Rumtopf recipe and a new sweater in a single day was now having to make do with watching TV and keeping track of her weight. That would be depressing enough for anyone!

Eckhart Tolle, author of *A New Earth*, would say that my ego was taking over my being. Just sitting, breathing, being should be enough. But my mind, or ego, isn't satisfied with that. According to him, ego is tied up closely with thought and one thing I could always do and was always proud of was my ability to think. Nothing that I tried with this mental/emotional work was working—yet. It doesn't seem possible to think your way out of chronic disease.

What I was really struggling with then was the concept of letting go, giving up. It could be a terrific stress release to just quit fighting. But did I have to resign myself to having MS and to being in a wheelchair in order to reach a state of acceptance? And is acceptance of this disease and my situation crucial to my future? These are questions that I continue to ask to this day. I've tried for a long time to find a compromise between accepting my situation and fighting my situation. How do I accept this disease and yet keep hoping for a cure? How do I keep fighting against my situation and at the same time, embrace it? I spent that early winter of 2014 in a dark place, lifted out solely by my painting efforts. Sitting in my wheelchair, looking out at the snow-covered fields through the large windows in our sunroom, I was physically comfortable and spiritually wrecked. I read a lot, thought a lot about my life, and I started to write, again. I have a friend who is in a wheelchair and who does very little in a day. Carol has lost the use of her hands and finally I decided that since I still have my hands, I need to use them. I produced a lot of pastel drawings that winter, learning to blend the pastels into the colours I saw around me, which were admittedly muted in January, and I spent time writing, noting down my thoughts and philosophies. Who knows, I thought, someday the kids might want to read this.

I struggled along and tried my best to make peace with my situation, having no idea at all of the changes that 2015 would bring to my life. Is there not a saying that "It is always darkest before the light"? I vaguely remember reading that somewhere and it does seem to be true. There was a hint that 2015 was going to be a brighter year on New Year's Eve. Once more, I was dancing. This time it was thanks to Angela.

New Year's Eve, 2015, we were at a ski club fundraiser and the band was good. I was sitting in my wheelchair, tapping my fingers in time with the beat of the music when Angela got up from the table and said, "Come dance with me." She walked and I wheeled up to the dance floor and both of us twisted and gyrated in time with the music. I, of course, could only move from the waist up but it still felt great to be moving in time with the beat. Angela didn't let the fact that her partner was female, let alone in a wheelchair, bother her at all and she seemed to enjoy the dance as much as I did. My recent past had been full of wins, like my painting and the new house, but it also had been full of losses: my job at Curves, my mobility and continuing attacks of depression. That night though, when the music once again took over my heartbeat, I felt something shift. I was ready to take on the new year and whatever it would bring.

Repairing and Renovating

*Acceptance doesn't mean resignation; it means understanding
that something is what it is and that there's got
to be a way through it.*
—Michael J. Fox

The brightness of 2015, rung in that New Year's Eve dancing with Angela, actually began because of a conversation I had in the summer of 2014. Tom and I went to visit Mom and Dad's neighbours, a couple who live at Rose Lake. The wife, who is my age, had just been diagnosed with multiple sclerosis and the couple were trying to figure out how to deal with their new situation. Tom and I talked about the realities of living with MS from our point of view, as patient and caretaker, and about different coping strategies. They told us about her visits to naturopaths and her desire to try a strict eating plan. She had in mind a particular clean diet, a healthy diet, a diet to beat MS. Like so many of us, I thought, she is in denial at the start of this journey. She'll soon learn that she can't beat MS. No one can.

"So what can you eat?"I asked politely.

"Kale and water." They grinned at us. We all laughed. I despise green vegetables and the little I knew of kale: it was green. Aside from saskatoon berries, I also dislike most fruit and am really a meat and dairy eater with lots of grains thrown in. My German background and natural inclinations lead me to eat breads, cakes and cookies, with butter and ice cream. That clean, healthy diet we ate at Sanoviv—the strictly no-sugar and restricted carbohydrates diet—had been the least pleasant part of that trip for me.

About a month after our visit to Rose Lake, I got a link to a YouTube video from this couple in a friendly email. The link was to a TedX talk called "Minding Your Mitochondria." The presenter was Dr. Terry Wahls. Out of curiosity, I watched the video. Dr. Wahls claimed to have cured herself of progressive multiple sclerosis by changing her diet. She had gotten out of her own wheelchair and back on her bicycle in the space of a year, simply by eating the nutrients her body needed to heal itself and by doing exercises as she healed. She extolled the virtues of vegetables, fruits, seaweed and fermented foods. My first thought was, Yuck! There were copious amounts of kale involved in this diet. I wished her well, but I remained deeply skeptical. All the doctors I had seen over the years, including neurologists, had repeatedly told me that there is no cure for MS.

There is no cure. MS is a progressive disease and it only gets worse with time.

That summer I chose to ignore the hope held out in that unappealing diet and, instead, resigned myself that MS is a progressive disease and I could not get any more relief from it. I was simply tired and I now wonder if I had actually stopped fighting. Fatigue and depression combined made it feel too hard for me to keep smiling. I was in a wheelchair, I was unhappy, and I was tremendously tired. Fear was a constant companion of mine, too. Some of my friends with MS were a bit more advanced with the disease than I was and I watched their trials and tribulations with trepidation. One of my friends suffered random seizures and was afraid to go on the strong medication that may or may not have helped her due to its severe side-effects. Another friend suffered from feet and ankles being so swollen she could no longer wear shoes.

As for me, I was started to notice my mind wandering off without me. This was another MS-related symptom and there is a term for it: brain fog. I caught Tom giving me exasperated glances as he patiently explained a concept to me. I knew from his expression that he had explained it to me before, maybe even as recently as the day before. There is a bright side to this, I tried to joke to myself: I can reread a favourite book or watch a favourite movie and it's like the first time I read the story or saw the film. Everything is new again.

Nevertheless, desperate to find a boost from somewhere, anywhere, I called the Mental Health Services people in Williams Lake and two intake workers came out to assess me. Shortly thereafter, I got an appointment with a mental health counsellor. Talking with her didn't help. It wasn't the answer—not for me, anyway. I knew deep down I would have to find my happiness in other ways: maybe in my painting or writing or in quiet moments with Tom; or even in passing conversations with my children, who make me so proud.

By the end of my bout with the flu that October, I had decided to give this diet thing a try. Being unable to move my legs scared me enough to snap me out of my deep lethargy. I rolled myself over to my computer and searched for Terry Wahls on YouTube and watched her video again. Then I went to Google. Dr. Wahls had now written a book and it was due to be released shortly. I called the bookstore in Williams Lake and ordered a copy.

On New Year's Eve, I danced with Angela and remembered how much joy I could still derive from my body. And on January 1, 2015, I read my copy of Dr. Wahls' book and I committed to the new diet and exercise protocol—kale and all. It was tough. God, it was tough. I could eat from basically four food groups: vegetables, meat, fruit and nuts. My German upbringing full of grains and my sweet tooth (candies, chocolates, sugar) rebelled and I spent the first four days on the toilet as my bladder wouldn't stop emptying itself. I learned later that that's what happens when you are "de-toxing."

In her video, Terry Wahls challenged people to try the diet for 100 days and see how they feel. I started counting days—days until I could eat bread and chocolate and get out of the bathroom. Plus, I felt lousy: I ached all over and was tired. I took the Medical Symptoms Questionnaire (MSQ) in the Wahls protocol book and scored a whopping 125 points. A normal, healthy person apparently scores about 10, or less. I was one sick person.

Then, things changed. After about the first week I noticed I had incrementally more energy and the world looked a little brighter. My MSQ score dropped by twenty points. The chronic, dull pain in my joints was gone. I decided I could hang in there and stay with the diet, at least for another week. And, best of all, I was finally off the toilet and out of the bathroom. It went like this for me, week after week, with small positive changes brightening my world. After about five weeks, I decided to try using my walker again and I got out of my wheelchair. I stopped napping throughout the day and took an interest in the world outside the house. Tom and I even talked about possibly taking a month-long holiday in May, in Australia! I stopped counting diet days and started looking forward to the future.

Before I knew it, it was May, and Tom and I *were* heading to Australia! I had been on the diet for over four months and it no longer seemed like a chore, especially because the benefits were so obvious. Whether it was the diet, or the return of my fighting spirit that made me feel better emotionally, I don't really know. I just know my compulsion to fight has proved to make me happy, in itself, in the past.

We went to Australia with my walker and we toured the east coast for three weeks in a rented caravan or motor home. Then we flew to Perth and visited friends for a week. We ate a lot of fresh fruit and vegetables and I continued to avoid gluten, dairy and sugary products. My spirits improved even more and my eyesight even sharpened. Life suddenly looked pretty good again.

Australia is a vast and diverse country. When we landed in Sydney, we immediately headed south along the coast. I was jubilant that the fifteen-hour-long flight hadn't sapped my energy as it would have, pre-diet. I was fully awake and aware of the ocean rolling in on the beach in our first campground south of Sydney and I loved the friendly, heavily accented Aussie voices coming from other caravans. By the time we got to Melbourne, I was even more confident in my improved health. Melbourne is a large and busy city. I was able to spend an entire day with Tom in Melbourne, walking the sidewalks with my walker, riding the buses and admiring the sights. An entire day without a nap would have been unthinkable a few short months ago.

I took hundreds of photos while we were in "Oz," and filled a thick album with them when we got home.

One of my favourites is a photo that Tom took. It shows a slim-faced, bright-eyed woman wearing a captain's hat as she pilots a paddlewheeler along the Murray River. Yup, that was me! I was fully living the life of a tourist and loving it!

I think the favourite part of Australia for both Tom and me, though, was the outback. We spent about four days driving through rust-red, sandy hills under a piercingly blue sky, along a road that ran straight without a single curve in it for those entire four days. The whole time we watched for kangaroos, rejoicing when we saw one of the energetic creatures bounding away through the grey-green, spiky brush beside the road. We also saw countless wild goats in colours ranging from all-black to pure white, emus that looked like overinflated, feathery beach balls on pogo-stick legs, and sheep. Sheep, sheep and more sheep. It wasn't until we left the outback and turned north that the sky filled with cockatoos and wild, white parrots. I remember the New England area, inland of Brisbane, as being old-country beautiful and reminding me strongly of Europe with its rolling, bare, green hills, dotted with dark clumps of conifers.

By the time we got to Rockhampton, our most northerly point on the trip, I was posing for a photograph beside the Tropic of Capricorn marker with my cane. It was the first time in two years that I was holding onto just a cane for support.

We flew to Perth and spent a week with Rod and Dorothy O'Dea, new friends we had met on the Mediterranean cruise. Dorothy and Rod toured us around southern Australia and helped to fill my photo album and my mind with pictures of crashing surf, seventy-metre high, shaggy red-barked karri trees and brilliant blue skies. Rod even arranged for us to see an Australian rules football game, knowing that Tom and I enjoy watching that sport. That day in particular, I found myself *walking for fifteen minutes with my walker* to get to the stadium. This woman did not need a wheelchair anymore! The O'Deas promised to come visit us in their turn in 2016 and we came home from Australia feeling very happy with our grand adventure.

By the time we came home in June, I stopped using the walker when I went to Williams Lake for groceries, relying instead on just my cane. Then I went back to Curves, but this time as a member.

Two months later, that August, my MSQ score was around thirty. I was still using a cane and, unfortunately, leg braces on each leg. Foot drop was still a real threat to me. When I was tired, I still tripped easily and fell so the leg braces were necessary. My bladder was also more active than I would've liked and I continued to be very intolerant of heat. Heat intolerance and my addiction to sugar and ice cream made summer a real challenge. I suspect that I didn't help myself any because I would often give in to the temptation of Dairy Queen Blizzard treats but in my defence, I will say that when you're feeling better, it's easy to fall back into old habits. At that point in time I was hoping strongly that my leg braces and cane could join my wheelchair in retirement by the end of the year.

I stuck with that diet, modified slightly to accommodate my taste for sugar. As a result of my inclination for sweets, I think, the great advances I noticed earlier in 2015 slowed but I still loved my new energy and willingness to tackle things. That fall, I started a new company and began offering editing and proofreading services, based on my long experience as a writer and self-editor. My first job, besides helping Ann by proofreading a grant application and some poems, was to ghost-write a book. Also in 2015, I went back to work for the Chamber of Commerce—but this time as a freelancer who writes business profiles for the chamber newsletter. This means I still interview business owners, but I don't go pale when faced with a flight of rickety stairs and a dubious handrail anymore. Instead, when I'm setting up the interview appointment, I tell the businessman or woman that I am handicapped and I request that the interview location be on the main floor of the business if there is no elevator accessibility to their office. Finally, I have the confidence to know who I am and not to be ashamed to ask for what I need.

Onwards and Upwards

Sometimes life knocks you on your ass…
get up, get up, get up!!! Happiness is not the absence of
problems, it's the ability to deal with them.
—Steve Maraboli

Now it's 2017, early March, a beautiful, early spring day down here in the Williams Lake Valley where Tom and I live. The heavy snow of this past winter has melted back and there are only drifts left in the hollows of the brown hills; drifts that look like misshapen white question marks. Two of the neighbour's horses just walked by, one reddish-brown and the other a black-and-white pinto. It is a beautiful day for a ride. Instead of riding, I'm sitting at my desk dreaming about riding. That's OK. My dreams are happy memories.

I am snacking on a bowl of nuts as I write this, filling my hunger with healthy protein rather than, say, sugary donuts. I've been watching what kinds of food I eat for over two years and while I cannot completely stop the progression of MS, the difference that the diet has made is undeniable. I have a lot to be grateful for. In the last couple of weeks alone, my balance has improved to the point that I am walking around the house without assistance. The difference that the Liberation Therapy made so many years ago, though more temporary than I would've liked, is also undeniable. My feet are warm and this morning I once again felt the warm water under the soles of my feet in the shower.

Life is good. The only downside to the new healthier, more assertive me these days is that sometimes I might be too assertive. If you ever park in a handicapped parking space in Williams Lake and you are not displaying a handicapped decal, you will find me leaning on my cane beside your car and I will explain in clear and loud tones that you are parked illegally. Also, if you happen to post a joke about "slow walkers" or God-help-you "handicapped people" on your Facebook feed, you will find a sharply worded rebuke from me telling you to get over yourself.

I have left instructions with my family that if I am suddenly struck down, they are to play Queen's "Another One Bites the Dust" at my funeral. I suspect now they may add the Munchkins' song from the *Wizard of Oz*: "Ding Dong, the Witch is Dead."

Life with MS has taught me many things over the past decade. I have learned to be humble and accept the help of strangers, like on that day in Rome when perfect strangers lifted me and my walker up over a curb and pushed me to the bus. I have learned to be patient when painting, trying to get a waterfall just right. I have learned to control my temper as there is no point in lashing out at non-believers in the Canadian medical system about procedures like the Liberation Therapy; only time will tell who is right on that front. Most of all I have learned to never, never, never give up. Onwards and upwards! I have multiple sclerosis. I will probably always have multiple sclerosis. I may always walk with a cane and leg braces. I don't care. Life is good. It occurs to me, finally, that I'm not a victim of this disease, or anything else. I am strong and resilient. I will survive.

Everything I've done to cope with this disease has been a learning experience. I've learned more about myself and what's really important to me as each year passes. I like to think I would have learned these things without MS, but I know it's sped up the process.

I am particularly grateful for the support of friends and family members, who continue to stand by me in my various endeavours and who never fail to cheer me up. Ann Walsh, in particular, makes me laugh in spite of myself when she recalls some memory of our shared past in the writers' group. Just the other day, she remarked how she had to often tiptoe around thorny subjects, specifically those related to MS, in fear that I might bite her head off if she mentioned it. Both she and Angela were my first customers when I started up my editing company last year. My friends, my husband and my children have my back, as do my parents. The other day, arriving at my parents' house, I found a newly installed grab-bar beside the back door, mere days after mentioning I was having difficulty struggling up their back steps.

On a brilliant early spring day like today, in the light sunshine under a bluebird sky, I celebrate everything that I am and that I still have. I sit at my desk—I still have that rock that Tom gave me that autumn day on the ranch so many years ago—and I write, and I take strength in the fact that I am a writer. I am a writer and a wife and a mother and I am my own person. I take pleasure in the horses that reside on my writing desk behind my computer. One of them is a lovely brass horse that I traded a painting for and one of them is a fat, little overstuffed horse that I was given at Spruce Meadows when Tom and I went to watch the Masters Jumping Tournament last fall.

Somehow, horses continue to be a part of my life even though my life has changed. I now use a wheelchair only when I want to, and last fall I used a wheelchair to propel myself around the vast grounds of the Spruce Meadows facility. From my comfortable perch in the handicap-accessible section of the viewing stands, I watched gorgeous, shining horses fly over jumps, towers and even ditches and I breathed in the throbbing vibrancy in that air with pure joy.

Gardening too, continues to be part of my life. Last fall, in 2016, we bought a Tower Garden, which is an indoor hydroponic system for growing whatever you want to grow. I think Tom initially thought it would be for lettuce but he was not too surprised to find sturdy yellow- orange nasturtiums and marigolds growing in it. We have been married for thirty years this coming June and very little that each of us does surprises the other partner any more.

We are planning another holiday this summer; probably we'll do another cross-Canada trip and I'm so grateful we can both still travel. Here at home, soon, I'll start seeing the hummingbirds back at the feeder and the first coreopsis and dandelions will start blooming. Our resident gophers will pop up from their burrows in front of our sunroom windows and we'll see how many babies they have with them. The long winter is almost over. I anticipate spring knowing that I will be able to greet it with enthusiasm, and energy, and gratitude. It is a long time since that May day when Tom drove me to the neurologist's appointment in which I first had my MS diagnosis confirmed; I still remember looking through the car window that day. The view then was much as it is now: thickly treed hills with patches of rolling grassland on their sides and in meadows at their feet. The only difference is that now I look at these hills with a full appreciation of their beauty. There is no shadow of fear hovering over my thoughts today. Tom's calm presence and the beauty of the land gave me great comfort that day. And they do now, too. My life is, in many ways, no less uncertain, but it is still beautiful, and it is still mine.

Acknowledgements

MS is not a solitary journey; neither is a life lived in the midst of family and friends. While there are many people in my life and my MS journey who have helped me along and who truly deserve a "thank you," there are some people who particularly stand out.

Ann Walsh, friend and writing mentor extraordinaire—your support and friendship over the years has meant more to me than I can ever tell you.

Angela Sommer and Verena Berger—thank you, thank you for the visits, the laughs and the kindnesses you've shown me over the years.

Bernie Suski—once you told me you loved me and I asked if you would still love me when I was in a wheelchair. That truly puzzled you and you asked me, "Why wouldn't I still love you?" That set my world right again, that day. Thank you, and I love you, too.

Chuck and Inge Wiggins and Barb Wiggins Koch—aka Dad, Mom and Bup, thank you for always having my back and encouraging me to keep on keeping on.

Ben, Sam and Lexie Redl—thank you for being you and for making me so very proud over the years. You have made my world a brighter one.

And finally, Tom Redl—it's been quite a ride and I couldn't have done it without you. You've been with me every step of the way; you've been my support, my encouragement and my number one cheerleader. I love you with all of my heart.

Extra thanks: Ruth Daniell, my sharp-eyed editor, thank you for taking a mass of words and nailing them to a timeline so that my thoughts make sense. Vici Johnstone at Caitlin Press, thank you for taking a chance on this story and making my dream of a published book come true.

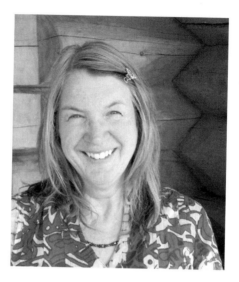

HEIDI REDL lives and writes with multiple sclerosis in Williams Lake, BC. Her columns and stories have appeared in *Canadian Cowboy Country* magazine, in the MS Kamloops chapter newsletter, in *Canadian Geographic* and in *MacLean's* magazines. She continues to write, to teach writing, and to struggle against the effects of MS in her life with the help of her husband, Tom, and her family and friends.